W9-AOE-936

METABOLISM.COM

Discover the Secrets to Effective Weight Loss or Weight Gain, Thyroid and Diabetes Treatments, Hormone Therapy and More

Gary Pepper, M.D.

Founder of Metabolism.com

METABOLISM.com

METABOLISM.COM: Discover the Secrets to Effective Weight Loss or Weight Gain, Thyroid and Diabetes Treatments, Hormone Therapy and More

© Copyright 2012 by Metabolink, Inc.

Disclaimer

Metabolism.com (owned and operated by Metabolink, Inc.) provides public access to a wide variety of well-informed opinions on nutritional and wellness issues. Our featured experts are not employees of Metabolink, Inc, but are independent practitioners of their chosen fields who have come to Metabolism.com to interact, help and teach. We do our best to make sure the credentials claimed by our featured experts are valid but cannot guarantee them. We encourage all visitors and members to take care to assure themselves of the validity of the expert's credentials, particularly if considering purchasing personal services from them.

The content and other information presented both in this Book ("Metabolism.com") and on the website Metabolism.com are for educational purposes only and should not serve as a substitute for medical counseling. If you are considering starting any diet, treatment, wellness or fitness program advocated within this Book or by one of the contributors to Metabolism. com, consult your physician or other health care provider to determine if it is right for your needs. Do not start a diet, treatment, wellness or fitness program if your physician or health care provider advises against it.

Users of this book agree that Dr. Gary Pepper (author), Metabolink, Inc. or its affiliates, subsidiaries, officers, directors, employees, agents, consultants, content providers, partners or suppliers ("Released Parties"), shall not have any liability to you under any theory of liability or indemnity in connection with your use of this book, ("Metabolism.com"). You further agree to hereby and forever release and waive any and all claims you may have against any Released Parties for any and all claims, causes, damages or losses under any theory of liability (including attorneys fees and associated costs and expenses) arising from your use of this book. Notwithstanding the foregoing, should your claim arise from a purchase made on or through our store, our total damages shall not exceed the cost of the product or service purchased (less shipping and handling). No representations or warranties of any kind whether express or implied fitness for a particular purpose or merchantability are made by us, regarding this Book. We will not be liable to you for any damages, including, direct or indirect, special, incidental, consequential or punitive damages even if we have been advised of the possibility of such damages. Void where prohibited by law.

Users of this book as well as the internet website metabolism.com and affiliated media managed by Metabolink, Inc. such as those found on Facebook and Twitter agree to be bound by the Terms and Conditions of Use found at: http://www.metabolism.com/2008/09/06/terms-conditions-service-agreement. A copy of these Terms and Conditions of Use can be obtained by requesting them by mail along with a self addressed stamped envelope, from Metabolink, Inc. 211 Anhinga Lane, Jupiter, Florida 33458.

PRINTED IN THE UNITED STATES OF AMERICA

Cover and interior design: Adina Cucicov, Flamingo Designs
Photography by Bryan Pepper

ISBN 978-0-9848727-0-1

In Tribute to Richard L. Neubauer, M.D., 1950-2011

For his life dedicated to providing care to those in need. For serving his profession, and his appreciation of nature. And for his love of his family and friends. He will always be a role model for those striving despite adversity, to be a positive force in this world.

Acknowledgements

In 15 years operating Metabolism.com I had the pleasure of working with many skilled professionals. I want to thank them all for contributing information and support to the website visitors. The following is a list of those providing the most service over these years, not necessarily in order of their importance: Robert Pastore, Ph.D; Theresa Davis, M.S., R.D.; Jennifer Schwallie, R.D.; Kimberly Russell, CN ; Brian Dean, R.D.; Sharon Linfante, CN, ; Maya Sarkisyan D.O.M., C.Ht., M.CS.; , Astrid Matthysse, R.D.; Beth Ellen DiLuglio, M.S., R.D., CCN.

I also want to thank Karen Vieira, M.S., Ph.D. and her talented staff at The Med Writers, for their help organizing, editing and completing this book. Without them I could not have undertaken this project.

I also thank Chris Drazek, owner of HauteProspect.com LLC, who over these last years has been the webmaster at Metabolism.com. We have weathered many challenges including attacks by hackers and being mauled by Google's Panda algorithm. The technical side of the

Internet has constantly shifting currents and his advice and assistance has kept Metabolism.com from disappearing under the electromagnetic waves like so many other small, independent websites.

METABOLISM.com

About The Author

Reaching and maintaining a healthy, desirable metabolism takes more than hard work—it takes knowledge. I've been proud to share my endocrinology and nutrition expertise with all the readers and members of Metabolism.com and now with you so you can look and feel healthier and happier.

Gary Pepper, M.D.; Board Certified by the American Boards of Internal Medicine, and Endocrinology and Metabolism. Dr. Pepper is the Founder and Editor-in-Chief at Metabolism.com. He received his medical degree from the Tufts School of Medicine in Boston and completed fellowship training in Endocrinology and Metabolism at Mt. Sinai Medical Center in New York City. Before joining the Palm Beach Diabetes and Endocrine Specialists, where he has practiced since 1996, Dr. Pepper served as Chief of the Division of Endocrinology and Metabolism at Lincoln Medical Center in the Bronx and later as the Associate Chief of Medicine at Brooklyn Hospital Center, director of the hospital's Diabetes Treatment Center, and Clinical Associate Professor of Medicine at New York University School of

Medicine. In recognition of these accomplishments Dr. Pepper was selected as one of the top 100 physicians in New York City by New York Magazine. He is also a featured expert with CNBC and iVillage on the topics of diabetes and endocrinology.

Table of Contents

Introduction

"I am at a total loss as to how to lose weight! Five years ago, I became chronically fatigued and had lots of other symptoms that led me to believe that I had an underactive thyroid. My doctor tested me and declared that I did not, and suggested that I should exercise more. My symptoms continued, and I began to gain weight at an alarming rate. I went back several times, presenting with hypothyroid symptoms, and he finally admitted that I was 'borderline hypo with a TSH over 5,' but 'we don't treat that.'

I lived the next two years with debilitating symptoms and weight gain that I simply could not control with diet and exercise. By the time I found a doctor who was willing to treat me, I had gained over 50 pounds and had developed fibromyalgia as well. Even then, it was difficult to get treatment, but finally he relented. Now my TSH is below 1, and my fatigue is not quite as debilitating; however, my weight loss efforts are dismal. I know that my metabolism is very slow—because my

temperature in the morning is usually under 96°. I've been on Atkins for six months now, keeping my carbs under 20 grams a day and relying on lots of fiber to keep me from being terribly hungry, but I've only managed to lose about 13 pounds. I know there has to be help for me, but I just don't know what to do.

Five and a half short years ago I weighed 140 pounds, had energy to burn and felt great, and looked pretty good too! Now I weigh 180 pounds, live with chronic pain and fatigue, and I'm unable to work. I've done a huge amount of research into hypothyroid and all the problems it causes—and bringing my TSH down has brought my glucose, triglycerides and cholesterol down, but not my weight. I am fearful of developing diabetes and really need help. I take Armour Thyroid, which has been much better for me than Synthroid was, but still I am startled and upset when I see a picture of myself looking fat and puffy instead of toned and slim. Please help me!"

Leslie

"I gave up smoking just one week ago, which is great BUT already the weight is piling on. As a 50-year-old female I'm not sure I want this weight gain. I exercise and watch what I eat. It seems like my metabolism has come to a grinding halt. Could smoking be the better option?"

Jean

"I am 40 years old and a Type 1 diabetic (insulin pump dependent). I work in a very fast-paced environment and get a lot of exercise, but I am tired all time and no matter what I do I cannot remove any weight. I am at around 232 pounds and would like to lose some weight to feel better and more energized without the stress and feeling of being tired all time. I need some advice, not only for better health, but for better control of my diabetes too. Any help will be greatly appreciated."

Bibis

"I have tried lots of different ways to gain weight. I am a 21-year-old male. I have been trying to gain weight for roughly four years now and all I've managed to do is lose weight. I am currently 113 pounds and even though I have probably been smaller, I feel the worst I have ever felt. I always get comments off people calling me skinny, and people are always saying to me: 'Eat something.'

As I work evenings, I don't have a normal routine diet. I wake up around 11am, and then eat either a banana or a chocolate bar. I go to work at 1pm, and between 1pm and 4pm I snack on junk food, normally chocolate. At 4pm I will have my first meal of the day. This almost always contains fries. But I do mix it up with different sides, either pasta, curry, sausages, or either gravy or beans. I normally have an energy drink with the meal. Between 4pm and 6pm I will snack again on either chocolate or chips. At 6pm I will have another meal, though *this varies hugely, as it depends what is on offer at the place I eat. I finish work at 9pm and return home. Sometimes I will have another meal with my other half. If so, it's normally take-away food.*

I do work all the time (so it feels). I have a very busy job work-ing in a factory-style environment, so I do burn off a lot of cal-ories during the day. As I've said above, I've just had enough of being the way I am and don't know where to go from here. I'm due to go for blood tests next week. But I highly doubt they will come back with anything. They will just tell me to eat more, like everyone else does."

Chris

Every day I meet people like Leslie, Jean, Bibis and Chris in my endo-crinology practice as well as on the message boards of Metabolism. com. These people come to me at their wits end, having tried every-thing and seen numerous doctors to get to the root of their problem, only to be told that the problem is them and their decisions. Howev-er, many times this isn't true. The problem can be their metabolism. And unfortunately, despite this fact, many endocrinologists (doctors who specialize in hormones and the glands that make them) are still unable to help.

When I became an endocrinologist in 1981, I was truly excited about the field. At the time it seemed as though the science of endocrinol-ogy was expanding rapidly and new discoveries were on the horizon, particularly with regard to the way hormones affected the brain, mood and the immune system. Was I overly optimistic!

During my fellowship at Mt. Sinai Medical Center in New York City my boss, Dr. Dorothy Krieger, was making exciting discoveries about how endorphins and other brain chemicals are produced and used in the circuits of the nervous system, functioning as powerful signals for hormone release, pleasure and reward. But now, more than 30 years later, there hasn't been any significant medications developed that take advantage of these discoveries. Instead of being able to help people with the vast advancements I envisioned at the beginning of my career, I often find that the field of endocrinology has barely budged in all of this time and has actually lost ground in some areas.

This is part of the reason why I started the website Metabolism.com in 1999. I wanted to share my knowledge and expertise on a wide range of problems related to metabolism, nutritional health and weight control, as well as conditions such as diabetes, thyroid disorders, high blood pressure and cholesterol management. Some of my opinions may be unpopular with other endocrinologists but my difference in opinion means I am able to help people who have been left feeling hopeless by their healthcare professionals.

Metabolism.com encourages people to discuss their own experiences and offer their personal advice, as well as giving everyone the opportunity to interact with our professional staff. This is because Metabolism.com (and this eBook) are not about us; they are about you—your questions, your stories, your triumphs and (sometimes)

your failures. Because even though the experts and nutritionists that contribute to the site have the education and clinical expertise, you have the real-life experience that demands a change from the status quo and can help inspire others to make changes for the better.

It is for this reason that I decided it was time to compile all of the advice about how to lose weight successfully, how to gain weight if you have a fast metabolism and how to treat thyroid and other hormone problems, from the blogs and forums of Metabolism.com into one easy-to-read and understand resource.

The first two sections will focus specifically on metabolism—what it is and why people have a "fast" or "slow" metabolism. Section three will focus on how you can increase or decrease your metabolism in order to move toward a more ideal weight, while section four will help dispel some of the misinformation that often surrounds discussions about metabolism. In the second half of this book, we will take a closer look at treatments for some of the most common metabolic issues, including thyroid disorders and diabetes, as well as other types of hormone treatment.

In the appendices at the end of the book, I included two complete examples of the personal nutrition profiles we developed at Metabolism.com. One of these profiles is designed for a member wanting to gain weight and the other for someone requesting help with weight loss. Each of these plans worth almost $100 (with on-line support) was specifically designed for the individual based on their food likes and dislikes, exercise capabilities and metabolic profiles. I include

METABOLISM™

them for free in this book to help readers learn what a truly valuable resource a professionally designed nutritional program can be.

It is my goal and my hope to give the members of Metabolism.com and everyone else who reads this eBook the practical information they need to achieve a healthy weight, abundant energy and lifelong health. Please read on to learn how your metabolism and hormones are the keys to achieving these goals. This is the resource and the support you have been asking for.

GARY PEPPER, M.D.
Board Certified by the American Boards of Internal Medicine, and Endocrinology and Metabolism
Founder, Metabolism.com

CHAPTER 1

What Is Metabolism?

"I've searched the web but found nothing that tells me how to distinguish if my metabolism is healthy. I've found plenty of ways to tell me how to improve my metabolism but nothing that explains what is normal. Are there outward signs that will tell you if your metabolism is healthy?"

Metabolism.com member

According to Webster's Dictionary, metabolism is "the chemical and physical processes continuously going on in living organisms." But when most people think about metabolism they focus on one specific process—the process that releases and stores energy from the food we eat. This is because this type of metabolism not only affects how efficiently your body burns fuel but also influences how easily our bodies gain or lose weight.

Turning Food into Energy

In simple terms, your metabolism is the rate at which your body breaks down nutrients from the foods you eat and converts them into a form the body can use.

After you've eaten a bowl of cereal or a sandwich, chemicals produced in the digestive tract, known as *enzymes*, break down all of the complex molecules that make up the food into smaller, more usable nutrients. Proteins are broken down into amino acids, fats into fatty acids, and carbohydrates into simple sugars like glucose. These nutrients are then absorbed into the blood where they are transported all over the body.

At this point the nutrients can be used in different processes. Amino acids are usually used to build and repair tissues, while glucose enters cells and is *metabolized* for energy. Any extra nutrients left over after these processes are generally stored in body tissues, especially the liver, muscles and body fat, and used for energy at a later date if the body needs it. (Think of it like a squirrel stocking up nuts for the winter.)

In this way, the process of metabolism really is a balancing act between two very different types of activities: (1) building up body tissues and energy stores, and (2) breaking down energy-rich nutrients, body tissues and energy stores to produce fuel that will power the body.

Anabolism, or constructive metabolism, focuses on building tissues and storing energy. During this process, small molecules are converted into larger, more complex molecules. For example, small molecules of glucose become larger, more complex storage molecules called glycogen. Amino acids are organized into proteins. And fatty acids are combined to create dreaded fat molecules. Anabolism is a very important process in the body, as it supports the growth and repair of cells and tissues and helps the body store energy so it can be used sometime in the future.

On the other hand, *catabolism*, or destructive metabolism, breaks down large molecules (mostly carbohydrates and fats) to release energy. We mostly refer to this energy burning as metabolism, even though this isn't the only type of metabolism. This is the process that fuels all of the activity in our cells and keeps our body running. It also provides the energy needed for anabolic, energy-storing processes, helps heat the body and enables our muscles to contract so we can move.

The Importance of Hormones

Hormones are chemical substances in the body that control and regulate the activity of certain cells or organs, as well as specific chemical and physical processes. Several important hormones are involved in controlling the rate and direction of metabolism:

The thyroid produces two important hormones called *thyroxine (T4)* and *triiodothyronine (T3)* that help determine how fast or slow the chemical reactions of metabolism proceed in a person's body. Every cell in the body depends on these two thyroid hormones to regulate their metabolism. The normal thyroid gland produces about 93% T4 and about 7% T3; however, T3 is about four times more powerful than T4.

Insulin, a hormone produced by the pancreas, is released when there is a lot of glucose in the blood. Insulin is often described as acting like a traffic cop because it directs glucose into the cells where it can be used for energy. Insulin also signals cells to store energy.

Glucagon is another important hormone produced by the pancreas. However, it is released when glucose levels in the blood start to fall because its job is to shut down the anabolic, energy-storing pathways promoted by insulin and turn on catabolic, energy-producing pathways. Glucagon also signals the body to start using stored energy reserves like glycogen as fuel.

Cortisol is a hormone produced by the adrenal gland, usually in response to stress; however, it also plays a role in metabolism. During times of nutrient shortage (fasting or skipping meals), cortisol stimulates the breakdown of fat reserves and muscle tissue so they can be used for energy.

Leptin is a hormone made by fat cells that circulates in the bloodstream before going to the brain. Leptin's main job is to tell your brain how much energy is stored in your fat cells. This means that as leptin levels rise, your brain knows that you have enough stored energy to keep your body going in case of a famine, so your appetite decreases and your metabolism increases. However, when your leptin levels fall, your body panics that it doesn't have enough energy stored for a rainy day, so your appetite increases and your metabolism decreases to help build up these backup energy reserves.

Human Growth Hormone (HGH) is produced by the pituitary gland. During childhood, this hormone fuels growth, but later in life it helps maintain tissues and organs, as well as play a role in protein, fat and carbohydrate metabolism. HGH encourages protein building (anabolism) in many tissues throughout the body. It also boosts fat burning by triggering triglyceride break down (lipolysis) as well as oxidation in fat cells. Finally, HGH helps maintain normal blood sugar levels. It has been shown to have anti-Insulin activity, which means HGH can stop insulin from stimulating the uptake of glucose by peripheral tissues so that it remains in the bloodstream.

Testosterone is the primary hormone produced by the testicles and promotes most of the masculine characteristics of the body. These 'secondary sexual characteristics' include development of the penis, increased muscle strength and mass, facial and body hair and male sexual function. Aging, as well as a number of medical conditions in men, can significantly lower testosterone levels, which can lead to symptoms such as loss of energy, depression, thinning of the bone (osteoporosis), loss of sexual interest and function, weight gain, and decreased muscle mass and strength, which indicates that testosterone plays a role in metabolism as well as sex drive.

Estrogen is the primary female sex hormone, and it is produced not only by the ovaries but by fat cells as well. Menopause, as well as a number of other medical conditions in women, can cause estrogen levels to plummet, causing hot flashes, night sweats, bloating, headaches, insomnia, fatigue, mood swings, depression, weight gain, anxiety attacks, aging skin, irritability, foggy thinking and bone loss. Women tend to gain weight during menopause because even though their estrogen production diminishes dramatically when they stop ovulating, their bodies still require some amount of estrogen to perform other metabolic functions. As a result, estrogen must be produced elsewhere. Since fat cells are able to produce estrogen, the brain sends messages to the body to preserve fat stores at all costs and to turn any excess calories into fat.

Role of Metabolism in Weight Loss or Gain

While understanding the basics of metabolism is important, most people really just want to know how these chemical processes affect their weight and health. In the end, it all really comes down to something known as energy balance when considering how metabolism affects weight. Simply put, energy balance describes the difference between the amount of calories you take in and the amount of calories you use. This is where calories come into play.

A calorie is a unit of measurement that describes how much energy a particular food can provide to the body. A cookie has more calories than a carrot, which means that it can supply more energy, but that's not always a good thing. When it comes to energy, more is not always better. This is because your body can only use a certain amount of energy, and the rest is put into storage.

Think of it this way. You only need a certain number of outfits to meet your clothing needs. However, if you keep shopping you will start to fill up your closet more and more. Eventually you will reach the point where clothes and shoes start spilling out every time you try to open the door. This is what happens to your body. You only need a certain amount of calories to meet your immediate energy needs. After that, your body will start storing energy in its 'closets' (i.e. the liver and muscles). However, there is only so much space, so if you eat too many calories they will start to 'spill out' as excess body fat.

When you take in more calories than you use, you are said to be in a state of *positive energy balance.* Don't be confused, this isn't positive as in good; it is positive as in 'increasing' or 'adding,' since this is how you start to gain weight.

On the flip side, when you are using more calories than you take in, you said to be in *negative energy balance,* which can lead to weight loss. The number of calories you use during a day is determined by a few different things: how much you exercise, the amount of fat and muscle in your body, and your basal metabolic rate (BMR). Your BMR is the bare minimum number of calories your body needs to keep itself alive. You can think about this as the amount of calories your body would have to burn to stay in bed asleep all day. (That big brain of yours doesn't stop working just because you've decided to catch 20 winks!) Most people refer to their BMR as their metabolism.

Your BMR is actually the largest factor determining your overall metabolic rate as well as how many calories are required to maintain, lose or gain weight. This means that if you had two people who were roughly the same height and weight eating the exact same diet and getting the same amount of exercise, the one with the lower BMR would tend to gain more pounds of body fat over time. This is what is often referred to as a 'slow metabolism.'

Is My Metabolism Healthy?

Everyone's metabolism is unique. Some people have a naturally fast metabolism, which means they burn up calories like a fiery furnace and can therefore eat more with little risk of weight gain. Other people have a naturally slow metabolism, which means they need to keep a closer eye on the foods they consume in order to remain at a healthy weight. Most people, though, fall somewhere in between these two extremes.

This means that as long as your body is able to break down the food you eat and convert it into enough energy to fuel your body, your metabolism is healthy. However, if you are significantly over- or underweight, this may be a sign that your metabolism is running on the fast or slow side. This could be the result of many different factors, some of which (like thyroid function) may need to be addressed by a doctor.

CHAPTER 2

What Makes Your Metabolism Fast or Slow?

"I recently spoke with a chiropractor about metabolism. He claims your metabolism is all based on your genes and family. I believe you can change your metabolism through exercise and diet. Can you explain please?"

Maskoliiko

Your metabolism is actually influenced by a combination of genetic, lifestyle and environmental factors:

- *Your age.* After you turn 20, your metabolism naturally slows by about 2% per decade. After age 40, it drops even more, decreasing by about 5% per decade. That's why many people who were thin in their younger years gain weight as they get older, even if they follow the same general dietary guidelines and exercise routine as before.

- **Your gender.** Men, because of their greater muscle mass and lower body fat percentage, generally have a 10-15% higher basal metabolic rate (BMR) than women.

- *Your weight.* The heavier you are, the higher your metabolism will be. For example, the resting metabolism of an obese woman is 25% higher than that of a thin woman. This is because the more you weigh, the harder your body has to work to keep itself running, even when you are resting.

- *Your muscle mass.* Muscle is a more active and energy-demanding tissue than fat. This means that more energy is needed to maintain these tissues. As a result, the higher your percentage of muscle (compared to fat), the faster your metabolism will be.

- *Your body surface area.* Body surface area (BSA) is calculated using both your height and weight. Researchers have found that the greater your BSA, the faster your resting metabolism. This means that tall, thin people tend to have higher BMRs. Also, if a tall person and a short person who weighed exactly the same both followed a diet designed to maintain the weight of the taller person, the shorter person could gain up to 15 pounds in a year!

- *Your diet.* Many people think that losing weight means eating less. However, when you don't get enough calories from your diet, your metabolism can slow by up to 30%. A healthy diet should consist of at least 3 balanced meals per day plus 1-3 snacks <u>or</u> 4 to 6 mini-meals per day. Following such an eating plan will help increase or maintain your metabolism much more effectively than an unhealthy, restrictive plan.

- *Your exercise routine.* An exercise program that includes aerobic and strength training activities helps improve your muscle-to-fat ratio, which keeps your metabolism high even when you are losing weight.

- *Rapid weight loss.* The process of weight loss itself slows down metabolism. Your body will never lose just fat when losing weight; your body also loses water and a little bit of muscle. Because of this muscle loss, your metabolism actually decreases a bit after weight loss. The more rapid your weight loss, the more muscle you lose. This is one reason why it's important to aim for slow gradual weight loss (about 1-2 pounds per week) because it will help preserve muscle to keep your metabolism up.

  Rapid weight loss also induces hormonal changes that can slow down metabolism. For example, levels of the potent thyroid hormone T3 decline during weight loss, which may explain why dieters find their weight loss plateaus after a brief period of success.

- *Smoking.* The nicotine found in tobacco products increases metabolism and energy expenditure, as well as reduces appetite. This may be why smokers tend to weigh less than non-smokers and often gain weight when they quit. Still, cigarette smoking increases insulin resistance and has been linked to central fat accumulation. As a result, smoking increases a person's risk of developing metabolic syndromes like diabetes, as well as increasing the risk of cardiovascular disease.

- *Your sleep patterns.* Insufficient sleep can seriously alter the levels of hormones linked to metabolism:

  - Insulin levels increase as a result of high blood sugar levels, causing the body to store more fat
  - Leptin levels decrease, which causes carbohydrate cravings
  - Growth hormone levels decline, affecting how the body regulates its muscle-to-fat balance
  - Additional cortisol is released, which can stimulate hunger

  Based on a study presented at the American Thoracic Society International Conference, women who slept for 5 hours a night were 32% more likely to experience major weight gain (defined as an increase of 33 pounds or more) and 15% more likely to become obese over the course of the 16-year study compared with women who slept 7 hours.

- *Your stress levels.* There are different types of stress, and their effects on your metabolic rate are very different as a result. For example, there is the metabolic stress of an illness, trauma or surgical procedure. These types of stressors actually increase our metabolic rate. However, the common stress we face in our daily lives will not increase metabolic rate, and evidence shows that it instead destroys our good intentions and resolutions to adopt healthy eating habits.

How we handle stress is the key. Some people use food as an outlet, to quell an emotional fire. This is a poor outlet and leads to weight gain. A recent study in the *American Journal of Clinical Nutrition* showed that when study participants are occupied with either a TV program, news article or mental problem, they consistently consume more food and a higher caloric intake than those not preoccupied or distracted while planning and eating meals.

The moral of this study is that our high-pressured lives keep us on "auto pilot," and we consume more calories than we need. Finding constructive outlets to stress, such as talking with friends, taking up a hobby, meditation, prayer, exercise, or any positive form of expression, can prevent the common distraction and self-medication with less than spectacular food choices during tough times.

- *Your exposure to light.* A research team from The Ohio State University discovered that mice exposed to a dim light during the course of a night for roughly a two-month period, gained 50% more body mass than mice exposed to a regular light-dark cycle. This is most likely because nighttime light exposure disrupts the natural rise and fall of the hormone melatonin. Since melatonin plays a significant role in metabolism, light exposure at night could disrupt the time animals choose to be active and eat and contribute to obesity.

- *Your genes.* The sad fact is that some people are just born with slower metabolisms than others.

The Role of the Thyroid

Probably the most important structure in your body when it comes to metabolism is your thyroid. The thyroid is a butterfly-shaped gland located in the front of your neck, just below the larynx (voice box). The main function of this gland is to control your metabolism by producing and releasing hormones like thyroxine (T4) and triiodothyronine (T3).

As I mentioned in the previous section, T3 and T4 are key players in regulating your resting metabolic rate. The more thyroid hormones that are produced and released, the higher your BMR will be. You might think that producing more and more thyroid hormones would be a good thing then. However, too much or too little of these hormones can cause serious health issues.

Hyperthyroidism is a condition that develops when the thyroid becomes overactive and produces too much thyroid hormone. Such high quantities of these hormones can actually double a person's BMR and can lead to symptoms such as severe weight loss, increased heart rate and blood pressure, protruding eyes, and goiter (a swelling in the neck caused by an enlarged thyroid gland). I need to point out that not everyone who has an over-active thyroid loses weight.

I estimate that about 1/3 of my patients with excess thyroid levels actually gain weight. My thought is that excess thyroid hormone stimulates the nervous system, and that can affect the appetite. After what would be a normal sized meal, these hyperthyroid people don't register the feeling of fullness (satiety) and so they continue to eat. This results in them consuming more calories than they can burn, leading to weight gain.

When your thyroid produces too little thyroid hormones, *hypothyroidism* can occur. This condition develops as a result of developmental problems, destructive diseases of the thyroid or thyroid under activity. The result is a very low metabolism (BMR) that may be 30-40% less than normal, as well as fatigue, slow heart rate, excessive weight gain and constipation. For infants and young children who don't receive treatment, hypothyroidism can lead to stunted growth and mental retardation.

Occasionally, a person's metabolic rate can also be affect by his/her nutritional status. Iodine, for example, is an essential component of the thyroid hormones that regulate metabolism. Therefore, without enough iodine, sufficient amounts of these hormones can't be produced, leading to sluggishness and weight gain. However, in countries like the United States where iodine is supplemented in various products (think iodized salt), this problem is relatively rare.

For people who have a very hard time losing or gaining weight despite following all of the usual medical and nutritional advice, making sure that your thyroid is functioning properly may be the first step to restoring the body's hormonal balance and reaching a healthy, desirable weight.

As you can see, while your metabolism may be influenced by your genes and family history, it is by no means carved in stone. There are still many ways to maximize the metabolism you have been born with—whether it runs fast or slow—in order to reach your ideal body weight.

CHAPTER 3

How to Increase or Decrease Metabolism

The practice of endocrinology deals with a lot of different conditions resulting from hormonal imbalances, of which weight problems is just one. Of course, in a public forum like Metabolism.com, questions and answers about weight gain and weight loss take up a large portion of the forum. But in my practice it is just one of the many conditions I treat.

Problems with Losing Weight

"I have a really slow metabolism and I was wondering besides exercise, is there anything I can do to speed it up, or should I go and see my doctor. I have tried to lose weight many times and have failed, what else can I do?"

Metabolism.com member

Exercise is probably the best way to increase your resting metabolic rate. This includes aerobic workouts to burn more calories in the short term, and weight training to build more muscles that will help boost your metabolism in the long term.

Since each pound of muscle burns more than 17 times as many calories as each pound of fat—even at rest—the more muscles you have, the higher your resting metabolic rate will be. This means that your body will be burning more calories just to keep your body alive.

Imagine putting in three days a week at the gym, pumping iron, and over time, noticing that you are burning more calories while you are watching TV or browsing the Internet!

Don't fall into the trap of thinking that strength exercises are just for increasing your size. You can do strength training and build more muscle without looking like a bodybuilder. The true payoff for doing strengthening exercises is that you will build more lean muscle mass, which will help you burn more calories throughout the day and speed your metabolism. How much your metabolism increases obviously depends on the amount of muscle mass you gain, but it is the only completely safe and natural method to increase your metabolic rate (unless exercise is not recommended due to a medical condition).

So instead of jumping on the treadmill or bike at the gym to lose weight and boost your metabolism, you should be hitting the dumbbells or machines. Even though, 30 minutes of aerobic exercise may burn more calories than 30 minutes of weight training, in the hours following the exercise, weight training has a longer-lasting effect on boosting metabolism. Therefore, supplement your strength training with an aerobic component to increase the amount of calories you burn and increase the success of your weight loss program even more, not the other way around.

The truth of the matter is, though, any movement has the potential to speed up your metabolism, including fidgeting (called non-exercise activity thermogenesis in scientific lingo, or NEAT for short). Every increase in body temperature of one degree increases your metabolic rate by 14% (eating protein appears to do the same thing naturally, by the way).

What and when you eat has a significant impact on your metabolism as well. Many people with slow metabolic rates think that increasing exercise and decreasing the amount of food they consume (usually by skipping meals) will be the key to meeting their weight-loss goals. However, when you starve yourself for more than twelve hours, your metabolic rate actually goes down by 40%! (That doesn't seem like the road to weight-loss success, now does it.)

When you skip meals, your body senses a dietary disaster and quickly goes into storage mode rather than burning mode. That's the primary reason why diets where you eat less often don't work. Your body panics about when and where its next meal might be coming from, so it slows metabolism into emergency-storing mode rather than a steady state of burning.

Small, but frequent, meals are the best way to keep your metabolism in high gear so that you can burn more calories overall. This is one reason why people who eat breakfast are on average thinner than those who skip breakfast. By starting their days with a well-balanced meal, they keep their metabolism running, which means that calories are more likely to be burned off before they can turn into fat.

Researchers from Georgia State University have found that snacks are also important for keeping metabolism levels pumped up throughout the day. They reported that when athletes ate snacks totaling about 250 calories each, three times a day, they had burned more energy than when they didn't snack. The study also found that snacking helped the athletes eat less at each of their three regular meals. The final result was a higher metabolic rate, a lower intake of calories and a reduction in body fat percentage.

Here are a few other diet tips to consider when you are trying to lose weight:

- Choose low-fat and nonfat milk, cheese, dressings, etc.
- Cut down on portion sizes by eating less than you are used to (try using smaller plates and bowls).
- Avoid having second portions.
- Avoid those tempting high-fat sauces and gravies, such as cream-based pasta sauces.
- Eat three balanced meals everyday and do not skip meals (this leads to excessive hunger and a tendency to snack and overeat).

- Eat slowly and take small bites, and remember to drink at least eight glasses of water a day.
- Limit the amounts of high-fat, high-sugar desserts you have.
- Remember to eat plenty of fruits and vegetables—these should be the bulk of your meals.

"I started working out 45 min a day, 5 times a week, and at first I would just starve myself, I would eat like an apple and some juice, for the day. I lost weight, but once the weekend hit, I totally caved, and I was like (oh well) I can just diet again once the week starts, but I would really like to know what food and how much of it I should eat."

Metabolism.com member

"Has anyone here tried using carnitine for weight loss?"

Metabolism.com member

Metabolism.com members also frequently want to know whether there are specific foods or supplements they can add to their diet to boost their metabolism and lose weight. But unfortunately while many products claim to boost metabolic rate, few actually do.

L-carnitine is found naturally in red meat and milk, is produced in the body when amino acids are broken down, and acts as an antioxidant. It is an important part of the process that transforms cellular fat into metabolic energy. The supplement has received mixed reviews, with some studies showing significant weight loss, increased muscle, improved cognitive function and less fatigue in patients who take L-carnitine as an oral supplement; while others have found no associated weight loss. L-carnitine, like many other supplements, has been shown to be potentially therapeutic in some disorders (for example, peripheral vascular disease and neuropathy), but toxic in high doses.

A powerful antioxidant in green tea known as EGCG (epigallocatechin gallate) is thought to have metabolism-boosting properties. In a study of 10 men published in the *American Journal of Clinical Nutrition*, researchers reported that 90 mg of EGCG and 50 mg of caffeine taken with meals boosted metabolism by 4%, while caffeine alone did not show a similar effect.

The Coca-Cola Company is currently taking advantage of this research by supplementing one of their new beverages, Enviga, with EGCG and caffeine. Calcium is also added to the mixture. Well-controlled scientific studies have shown a small metabolic increase in people consuming Enviga three times a day for several days. Another similar product is marketed by the Elite Company under the brand name Celsius. You may wonder if Dr. Pepper should be recommending other soft drinks and my answer is "only if they are good for you!".

While EGCG may boost metabolism slightly, it's not yet clear whether this effect would be enough to increase weight loss in the people consuming it. Therefore, it is probably better to drink green tea for its other health-giving properties (like preventing heart disease, cancer and diabetes) rather than to lose weight.

Very spicy foods are another popular recommendation for boosting metabolism. Some studies have shown that hot peppers and other very spicy foods can increase metabolism by about 20% for 30 minutes after a meal, but no one really knows if this extra burn can cause weight loss.

In a small study on Japanese women published in the *British Journal of Nutrition*, researchers found that red pepper increased body temperature and revved up metabolism following a meal. However, the greatest effects were seen when the red pepper was eaten with high-fat foods, which are also higher in calories, and not exactly the best diet for losing weight to begin with.

Another group of researchers reported in the *Journal of Medicine and Science in Sports and Exercise* that male athletes who added red pepper to high-carbohydrate meals boosted both their resting and active metabolic rates for about 30 minutes after finishing their meal. But there was no evidence this calorie burn continued beyond that.

There are many EGCG and red pepper supplements, as well as other weight loss products, available that claim to curb your appetite, melt away fat or boost your metabolism. Be aware, though, that using some of these without medical clearance and guidance may be extremely harmful and of course they may not even work.

Many patients and Metabolism.com users ask me why, after so many years of research, and such a great public need, there have been so few scientific advances and FDA-approved weight loss drugs available. With obesity and type 2 diabetes reaching epidemic levels in the United States, it is surprising that the FDA has been so slow to approve new weight loss medicines.

The answer is that the FDA is extremely cautious, for example, rejecting three new drugs designed to induce weight loss that performed well in clinical trials (Qnexa, Topamax and Lorgess) on the basis that they were too risky. With the number of potential customers for a weight-loss pill in the millions, even a very low probability of side effects or abuse is too high.

Rather than beat up on the FDA for being ultra-conservative, I try to put myself in the position of the Chairman of the FDA. As a Federal employee I would represent the government, and criticism of the FDA reflects very badly on the elected officials who gave me my job. Even as Chairman of the FDA, I depend on my job just like everyone else and if my boss gets a black eye I will get the boot and stand alone in the spotlight facing a lot of very public criticism. Why defend a controversial position when I can take the safe way out and say, "Denied!" Looking at it that way I don't blame the people at the FDA for rejecting a drug that could be abused or cause any harm what-so-ever.

Because of the system of drug approval in the U.S., I predict that it will be at least another 10 years before a medication for weight loss is approved by the FDA. As there is no magic bullet, we are left to pursue more natural ways of losing weight.

Your best bet for increasing your metabolism and keeping it high is to build muscle; snack on low-calorie, high-protein foods; and keep your body moving. However, if you have already changed your diet and exercise routine and still aren't losing the weight you would expect, there may be other factors that are keeping you from losing weight. Eating out, for example, could be holding you back.

Meals eaten outside your house often consist of larger portions and contain "hidden" extras (bread and butter, high-calorie desserts, fatty sauces, etc.). If you do want to eat out, there are some precautions you can take so you don't sabotage your weight-loss efforts:

- Avoid fried foods and cream- or cheese-based sauces.
- Ask for the breadbasket and butter dish to be removed from the table.
- Start your meal with a salad and low-fat dressing so you will be less hungry for the rest of the meal.
- Eat slowly and take small bites.
- Choose water, seltzer or diet sodas rather than regular soda, juices or alcoholic drinks.
- Share a dish with another person, or take half of it home for another meal.
- If you just can't resist dessert, share that too.

If you find and eliminate these hidden extras and still are finding weight loss a challenge, it would probably be beneficial for you to consult with a physician in order to rule out any metabolic or medical conditions. There are some endocrine disorders that can result in the inability to lose weight. Hypothyroidism is one such condition, and must be addressed by an endocrinologist. Please talk to your doctor to rule out any possible health problems.

> NOTE: Want more specifics? Even more recommendations on diet, exercise and dietary supplements to help your lose weight can be found in *Appendix 1* at the end of this book.

Problems with Gaining Weight

> *"I have a very high metabolism and I cannot gain weight. My energy level sometimes makes me feel worn out. Is there a way to gain weight/muscle that is healthy?"*
>
> **Metabolism.com member**

While many members of Metabolism.com struggle with low metabolism, fatigue and weight gain, there are also those who struggle with the exact opposite. As one member put it: "I eat like a pig. I exercise like a Marine, I hit the gym, but I never gain weight." For them, being underweight is as difficult to cope with as being overweight.

Riley writes:

> *"I have been trying for years to gain weight, and I have weighed 85 pounds now for 2 years, and I work at McDonald's and eat so much there (probably not good) but other than that I eat 6 or 7 meals a day and I can't even gain one pound and I'm so*

self conscious because of it...like I can't wear skirts or t-shirts or tank tops—I'm scared to. And everyone thinks I'm anorexic if they don't know me. But all I do is eat. I have to base my life around being so skinny, and I look so gross—even I think I look gross. I just want to look like all my friends—normal.

I am so stumped; it is upsetting and very frustrating trying to gain weight. My whole family goes up and down in weight very easily, and I can't even gain a pound. I can't fit into clothes from most stores, and I tend to wear baggy clothes because when I get made fun of constantly I really do just want to hide my body from everyone. Summer scares me...me in a two-piece bathing suit—I'm so self-conscious. I just can't take it anymore. And everyone is like: 'You're so lucky.' 'Oh my goodness, shut up I would kill to be that size.' And seriously you may think that, but I'm not normal looking; I'm not a nice size. It scares me and other people. I hate this soooo much."

Many people with high metabolisms make a concerted effort to gain weight by eating foods that are high in calories. But no one, even those struggling to gain weight, wants to gain fat. They want to gain *healthy weight*, which means increasing their lean body mass (muscle). Eating junk food all the time is not the way to do this. Junk foods not only make you feel tired and run down, but they could set you up for health problems down the road. Therefore, it is much better to try to gain weight in a more healthy way.

One of the first things to try is a supplement like *Boost* or *Ensure*. These don't fill you up, but have a lot of calories and are much healthier than junk food. Drink 2-3 per day after meals and you will almost certainly start to gain some weight.

Here are some other eating strategies that may help you increase your body weight:

- Eat high-calorie foods that are healthy. Choose a milkshake instead of nonfat milk, and avocados instead of cucumbers. For health reasons, choose mostly vegetable fats (olive and vegetable oils, nuts) rather than animal fats (butter, cream). Also try adding nuts (unsalted of course) to salads, cereals and shakes for an extra calorie boost.

- Choose low-fat dairy and lean meats most of the time. Dairy and meat products are a source of saturated fat, the type of fat associated with increasing the risk of heart disease. Although you're looking to gain weight, lean meats and low-fat dairy products are still a better option. Remember, though, low-fat *not* non-fat.

- Eat at least three healthy meals every day. Skipping meals robs the body of needed calories as well as leaving you more prone to snacking on unhealthy foods.

- Eat more food at each meal. Choose bigger portions, add extra fillings to sandwiches and use bigger drinking glasses, plates and bowls.

- Eat at least three snacks in between meals. Carry healthy foods like granola bars, whole-grain crackers and pretzels to eat on the run. Try snacking on a handful of nuts or olives in between meals. If you find that it's tough for you to eat three snacks as well as three meals a day, try drinking protein or yogurt shakes instead of snacking. For many people it's easier to drink their calories than to eat them.

- Add sauces and gravies to food. Cheese sauces on cooked vegetables increase the calories and provide flavor.

- Eat more peanut butter. Besides eating peanut butter sandwiches, add peanut butter to shakes, oatmeal or as a spread on fruit and veggies.

- Drink plenty of juices and milk throughout the day. This is a simple way to add calories without feeling full. Adding powered milk or instant breakfast powder to milk contributes extra calories.

"Hi, I am a 40 yr. old male, diagnosed with fibromyalgia and hypothyroidisim. I have weighed between 118 and 122 most of my adult life and have not been able to gain an ounce more. I eat like food is going out of style and it does no good, any advice would be much appreciated."

Metabolism.com member

Many members of Metabolism.com are interested in supplements or foods that they can include in their diet that will slow down their metabolism and keep their weight up. Gaining healthy weight (as opposed to fat), like losing weight, is a matter of restoring metabolic balance to the body. This can be achieved with the help of a balanced diet, and with supplements like L-carnitine. Yes, L-carnitine is also a popular supplement used to lose weight. How does this work? The key is that this supplement may increase muscle mass, while reducing fat tissue in the body. However, this has only been shown in a few studies, and has yet to be proven. Functional levels of L-carnitine are reportedly measured by various commercial laboratories found on the Internet. This type of test will show you if you have low levels of L-carnitine and if you could do with a boost.

Exercise may be the best way to increase muscle mass (and produce good weight gain) as it keeps the extra calories in your diet from turning into body fat and instead helps build muscle. This added muscle adds weight in the parts of the body where the weight should be.

The type of exercise you do is extremely important, though. You need to focus more on strength training, which builds muscle, rather than cardiovascular exercise, which predominantly burns fat. You need to work hard because you need to tear those muscles before they can repair themselves and become stronger. But be aware that there are two different kinds of repairs after spending time in the gym. When you feel tired and achy yet you know you can pull off more sets, that's called muscle fatigue. That's for endurance and toning, not muscle building. When you push the heavy weight until you literally can't move any more, this is called muscle failure. This is where you need to be. Keep in mind, though, you need to work towards muscle failure not muscle torture!

A Pleasurable Exercise Routine is a Must

A note of warning here! One of the most common causes of giving up any exercise routine is over doing it. Whether you want to increase your endurance, gain tone or add muscle, we must respect our body's limits. I like to think of working with the body as working with the family dog. Dogs work on the simplest principles of pleasure, pain and reward. So do the areas of the brain related to our body functions. If you want your dog to learn a new trick, using reward and pleasure are much stronger incentives than pain. Your dog will do anything to avoid the pain but come running for a treat. If you cause your body too much pain during exercise the next time you have to step on the treadmill or go to the gym, you are likely to find some other activity that needs doing or you may feel too "exhausted" to get started. Be gentle and go slowly with your exercise routine and find ways to make it fun and you will be much more likely to develop a lifelong healthy exercise habit.

Rest is equally essential for trying to gain weight since your body regenerates while you are asleep. Thus you need to keep regular sleep patterns. Getting sufficient uninterrupted sleep is also important.

Finally, work on keeping your stress levels under control. Stress can cause weight loss so it is a good idea to make time to reduce the amount of stress in your life. Consider everyday events and feelings that cause you stress and work on eliminating them, not for peace of body, but for peace of mind, too. Pilates, yoga, breathing exercises, meditation and a good self-image are all good sources of stress relief.

Don't beat yourself up if you don't see results right away. Be patient— gaining healthy weight isn't something that happens overnight. However, if you continue to lose weight or notice no improvements at all despite following these suggestions, it may be a good idea to check with a doctor in order to rule out any metabolic problems or other medical issues that may be causing your low weight. Consulting a registered dietitian can also provide better insight on the nature of the problem and result in more accurate recommendations that are better suited for your lifestyle and food preferences.

> NOTE: Want more specifics? More diet and exercise tips and a complete weight-gain program designed by the experts at Metabolism.com can be found in *Appendix 2* at the end of this book.

CHAPTER 4

Fact vs. Fiction—
Smoking and Weight Loss

"I have smoked for about 25 years and recently stopped. Now I am fighting weight gain. What can I expect and what can I do to keep the weight gain to a minimum? What is it that happens to the metabolism that causes the weight to go on so fast?"

Metabolism.com member

There is a lot of misinformation out there about smoking and weight gain. In fact, many people mistakenly believe that keeping weight off through smoking is worth the price they pay with their health. The biggest fact you need to know is: Not only will stopping smoking reduce your risk of cardiovascular disease, cancer and a host of other health problems, but quitting smoking will add an extra 2 to 4 years to your life.

Yes, quitting may be difficult, but with the right approach to eating/exercising it doesn't have to come at the expense of your waistline. And, according to many of our experts and members, it is well worth the effort.

The fact of the matter is that nicotine, the main drug in cigarettes, elevates your metabolism slightly by stimulating the central nervous system. However, when you quit smoking your metabolism doesn't slow way down, it simply returns to normal once the nicotine has been removed from your system. This difference is not very significant and you should adjust to it in a short period of time.

Therefore, while reductions in your metabolism may be a factor in post-smoking weight gain, it isn't the main culprit. Your eating habits are. First, smoking appears to ease feelings of hunger. This means that instead of eating to overcome hunger signals, many smokers light up. Secondly, your taste buds become desensitized because of the nicotine so food doesn't taste as good, making you eat less. Consequently, there's a tendency to eat more once you quit smoking, which is why weight gain is often experienced soon after a person quits smoking.

Not everyone gains weight after quitting, and the average weight gain for people who quit is less than 10 pounds. Gaining more than 10 pounds usually is an indication of over-eating.

Being aware of the problem in advance will help you avoid or minimize any potential weight gain. When people quit smoking their bodies have to go through some sort of rearrangement. Since food will start to taste better and you might experience depression when you quit smoking, food is an easy place to turn for comfort. Therefore, it is important to start adjusting your diet and exercise routines even prior to quitting in order to prepare yourself.

Here are some other suggestions from our experts and members to help minimize any potential weight gain after quitting:

- Choose a diet rich in fruits and vegetables, whole grains, lean proteins, low-fat dairy and heart-healthy fats.

- Have at least three balanced meals and one to two snacks per day that contain the foods mentioned above.

- Never skip meals. It leads to hunger and a tendency to snack on high-calorie foods.

- Try covering half your plate at lunch and dinner with watery vegetables (such as salad greens, tomatoes, broccoli, cauliflower, peppers, etc). Cover another quarter with lean meats, and the last quarter with whole grains such as brown rice, whole-wheat pasta, barley, etc.

- Eliminate sugary beverages such as soft drinks and juice from your diet.

- Limit or eliminate foods such as sweets, chips and pretzels, as well as alcoholic beverages from your diet.

* Keep fresh fruit and raw vegetables cut up in the fridge so they are handy when you need a snack.

* Keep busy to keep your thoughts away from food and smoking. Choose an activity that you enjoy (except eating) and do it more often.

* Engage in 60 minutes of vigorous physical activity 3—5 days per week.

* Always discuss any changes to your diet or activity level with your doctor before implementing.

Never let the fear of weight gain keep you from accomplishing your goal. With a little effort and determination you will succeed in not just quitting smoking but also avoiding weight gain. Just look at what Greg has to say:

> *"I hope what I am about to write will be an inspiration for those who are truly serious about quitting AND losing weight. I have now been almost five months without a cigarette (the longest I have EVER lasted) and unlike every other time I tried quitting, this time I FEEL it's for good. Truthfully, no temptations other than a quick subconscious glance (like noticing cleavage on a woman)!*

> *Every time I quit in the past, I gained at least five pounds, then lost it as soon as I started smoking again. This time I*

tried a different strategy overall and it has made a world of difference. Instead of making my goal 'quitting smoking and holding weight,' I made my goal far more ambitious: 'quitting smoking and losing weight, gaining muscle, and looking 100% better overall.'

I am now 42. About ten years ago (while I was still smoking), before I met my wife, I lost about 20 lbs (and 12% body fat) in four months by simply using a bodybuilder's type workout (3-5 set pyramid, every five days upper body and lower alternating), light-medium cardio two to three days per week, plus eating on the Zone Diet (40 Protein/40 Carb/20 Fat) five times per day. The results were so dramatic and so fast that one of my teachers at college thought I was sick or on drugs.

When I quit smoking in October, I started the same routine. At first, my goal was to hold weight only...not to gain. But now, four and a half months later, I went from 200 lbs to 184 lbs and over 29% body fat to under 22% body fat. Now that's not nearly as dramatic as the last transformation when I was 32 and smoking, but hell, at 42 and no longer smoking I am beating the monster and looking and feeling better every day.

Truth be told, if I was smoking and my metabolism was up, I'd probably be losing faster. But who cares, the fact is I'm clean of smokes and feeling and looking better than I did this time last year.

This isn't a pitch for supplements, a workout program, or any other BS. I am just saying that if you truly want to quit AND lose weight, it is possible even at 42. Just be smart about it AND totally committed. I think this time what made the big difference was making my mind up that I will settle for nothing less. Now, four and a half months into my quit, my goal is 170 lbs and 12% body fat. F#@k smoking! F$#k gaining weight! I want to breathe a full breath of air and see a six pack of abs in the mirror!

Anyone who tells you that gaining weight is the price of quitting is lying or, more likely, just doesn't know otherwise yet. Keep the faith!"

CHAPTER 5

Thyroid Treatment

As explained earlier, the thyroid is one of the most important glands in the body, controlling metabolism, protein synthesis and the function of other hormones throughout the body. The thyroid gland produces the hormones T3 (triiodothyronine) and T4 (thyroxine) from iodine and an amino acid, tyrosine, found in the food we eat. These two hormones work together to keep the body's metabolic rate within a narrow "optimal" range.

How Are T3 and T4 Regulated?

The key players that regulate the release of T3 and T4 are two structures located in the brain: the hypothalamus and the pituitary gland. If the hypothalamus receives signals that blood levels of T3 and T4 are low, it releases TRH (thyrotropin-releasing hormone), which then signals the pituitary gland to release TSH (thyroid stimulating hormone). TSH in turn triggers the production of T3 and T4 in the thyroid. Think of the hypothalamus and pituitary gland working together as a thermostat that tells the furnace (thyroid) to pump up or decrease the amount of thyroid hormone in the blood.

When functioning correctly, the two hormones (approximately 93% T4 and 7% T3) released from the thyroid are transported by the blood stream to the body's tissues. T3 is much more effective than T4, since T4 functions as a kind of storage molecule that can be converted into active T3 when needed. It makes perfect sense that such a powerful hormone (T3) is kept in its inactive form (T4) until required. Most T4 is eventually converted into T3 in tissues such as the brain, liver, kidney, spleen and muscles. However, this conversion process is not identical in all individuals, and varies because of genetics.

Most of the T4 and T3 in the body is bound up by carrier molecules such as thyroid binding globulin (TBG), which transports the hormones to their destinations. When they are being transported they are inactive. Only a very small amount of T3 and T4 is active because the body tightly controls how much active hormone is available. For example, when T4 levels in the blood are too high, TSH production from the pituitary gland (the thermostat) stops so that the thyroid is no longer signaled to make more T4.

Types of Thyroid Diseases

It is not surprising, given how important these hormones are for normal functioning of the body, that any disruption of the T3 and T4 balance has serious consequences. Overproduction or increased activity of these hormones causes *hyper*thyroidism, and underproduction or decreased activity causes *hypo*thyroidism.

Hyper- and Hypothyroidism

Most cases of naturally occurring hyperthyroidism and hypothyroidism are caused by an abnormal immune system response known as autoimmunity. The immune system consists of specialized white blood cells and the products they produce. Most important of these white cell products are antibodies that attack foreign proteins and cytokines, which are inflammatory molecules. However, autoimmunity occurs when the immune system starts attacking the body's normal, healthy "self" tissues rather than invading viruses or bacteria.

Hyper- and hypothyroidism often result when the immune system produces antibodies against the otherwise normal thyroid gland. The misdirected antibodies can result in either an under-active thyroid or an over-active thyroid. In either case the antibodies also cause the thyroid to enlarge into a "goiter," which is visible as a swollen neck. Hypothyroidism resulting from autoimmune attack is termed Hashimoto's Thyroiditis or Chronic Lymphocytic Thyroiditis, while autoimmune hyperthyroidism is Grave's Disease.

Autoimmune thyroid disease is strongly inherited, is almost 10 times more common in women and can come and go for no apparent reason. Additionally, in the same family one person may have Hashimoto's and another may have Grave's Disease. I have seen a Grave's mother deliver a baby with Hashimoto's.

It's also interesting to note that it's possible to swing from hyperthyroidism to hypothyroidism and more rarely hypothyroidism to hyperthyroidism. When Grave's disease transitions into hypothyroidism the process is sometimes referred to as thyroid burnout. When a formerly hypothyroid person develops Grave's Disease it is completely unexpected and can go undiagnosed for a long time. Although you won't find this term in the textbooks I like to call this the "Zombie Thyroid" because the thyroid comes back from the dead. My advice for those who suspect they have this condition is to remind your doctor that such things do exist. ("Beware the Zombie Thyroid" is a favorite line of mine.) In fact, Dr. Terry Davies teaches that autoimmune thyroid disorder should be seen as a continuum from hyper- to hypothyroidism and not as separate diseases. An individual with autoimmune thyroid disease is capable of moving anywhere within that spectrum over time.

Autoimmune thyroid diseases can be diagnosed with readily available commercial blood tests. The antithyroid antibody panel detects two different antibodies: the anti-peroxidase antibody and the anti-thyroglobulin antibody. If either comes back positive, the diagnosis of Hashimoto's Thyroiditis is confirmed. For Grave's disease a positive test for Thyroid Stimulating Immunoglobulin will make the diagnosis.

Autoimmune thyroid disease is also associated with other autoimmune diseases such as vitiligo (depigmented patches of skin), patchy hair loss known as alopecia areata, exophthalmus (thyroid-related eye disease), and more rarely rheumatoid arthritis, lupus, inflammatory bowel disease and Type 1 diabetes.

It is unclear why autoimmune thyroid diseases are so much more common in women. It is obvious that sex hormones play a role here. Could it be that estrogen provokes abnormalities of the immune system or can testosterone suppress abnormal immune cells? Both theories have support. Perhaps it is a combination of both. Something that occurred to me recently is that women also have an extra layer of fat under their skin. Research is now showing that fat tissue may cause inflammatory immune changes, but if this were the cause of autoimmune disease heavier people would show more autoimmune disease and so far, there does not appear to be a very strong association.

Thyroid Nodules

The term "nodule" (as it applies to the thyroid) simply means a bump or a lump. It isn't very doctorly to use terms like bump or lump so we say "nodule". Most thyroid nodules are harmless and an often-quoted statistic is that if you investigated the thyroid of 100 normal people, 50 of them would have a thyroid nodule or nodules.

The best way to detect and analyze a thyroid nodule is with an ultrasound. CT, MRI and PET scans will also show nodules within the thyroid, but the ultrasound is the most widely used and best characterized method. The other types of radiologic studies are overkill and usually unnecessary. Occasionally a thyroid "scan" may be needed, which uses radioactive iodine to clarify the function of the thyroid gland or thyroid nodule, but this type of study is being used less and less to investigate thyroid nodules.

A thyroid nodule may represent thyroid cancer and for that reason needs to be evaluated thoroughly. If the nodule is thought to have cancer potential an aspiration biopsy of the thyroid is then performed. The aspiration biopsy became widely used in the last 30 years and is a generally safe and easy procedure. In the early 1980's this type of test was usually only offered in large academic hospitals. As an Assistant Professor at Downstate Medical Center in Brooklyn, New York I published a paper with my collaborators in the mid 80s showing that aspiration biopsy could be adapted to local community hospitals. The procedure has now gained such wide acceptance that most endocrinologists perform the procedure in their own offices.

If the aspiration biopsy of the thyroid nodule is either suspicious or definitive for cancer, the endocrinologist is almost always going to advise that the thyroid nodule and most or all of the rest of the thyroid gland, be surgically removed. Fortunately, most forms of thyroid cancer can be cured by surgery and in some instances, require a follow up dose of radioactive iodine.

A major limitation of the thyroid biopsy is the frequent occurrence of an indeterminate specimen. The aspiration biopsy produces only microscopic pieces of the thyroid for analysis and sometimes the pathologist is unable to determine whether the available thyroid cells are cancerous or just slightly abnormal, non-cancerous cells. In the past year new technology using DNA analysis is enabling doctors to make better decisions about which cells are cancer and which are not. One company which provides this type of analysis, which I have started using in my practice, is Veracyte Corporation. My colleagues and I are waiting anxiously to find out how practical this approach is, and I should be updating Metabolism.com with progress in the near future.

Is Your Thyroid Nodule Hot?

A specific instance of a non-cancerous thyroid nodule with particular significance is the "hot" thyroid nodule. The hot nodule is an area of the thyroid composed of a single clone of thyroid cells behaving independently from the rest of the gland, over producing thyroid hormone. This area known as an adenoma, may exist for years before it reaches a point where the clone takes over the total production of thyroid hormone resulting in hyperthyroidism. This is different than autoimmune Grave's disease in which the whole thyroid gland is over producing thyroid hormone equally. Hot nodules are generally found in the older age group of patients and can have an insidiously slow onset easily over looked. Common findings include rapid heart rate, atrial fibrillation, weight loss, lethargy, mood changes, and tremor. These signs and symptoms mimic depression or cancer and can lead to many unnecessary diagnostic tests and treatments until the real cause is uncovered. Diagnosis is fairly easy because blood tests reveal excessive thyroid hormone levels, low TSH and a nuclear thyroid scan shows a typical single area of hyperactivity. It is the nodule's appearance on the thyroid scan as a solitary extremely bright area with the remainder of the gland turned off, which is the origin of the term "hot nodule".

Thyroid Treatments

> *"I have been suffering with hypothyroidism for 14 years now (10 years undiagnosed, 4 years insufficiently treated)…I fail to understand why the vast majority of General Practitioners don't get up to speed on this subject since so many of their patients are suffering from thyroid problems…"*
>
> **Metabolism.com member**

> *"I'm living in the UK and have been diagnosed hypo for 2 1/2 years. For the last 12 months I have been on 100mcg. I do not feel any better at all since starting treatment. If anything my symptoms have got worse—cold, fatigue, memory loss, dry skin, weight gain despite low appetite…"*
>
> **Metabolism.com member**

Given that multiple systems, organs and regulatory mechanisms are involved in keeping the delicate thyroid hormone system in balance, it is not surprising that treating thyroid problems is not as easy as just taking a never-changing dose of a T4 pill.

The wide spread dissatisfaction with the treatment of thyroid problems is in part caused by the fact that many doctors treat thyroid problems with a one-size-fits-all approach. For example, you may not feel well even though you are on thyroid medication, but when your blood test results come back, you are told by your doctor that your thyroid hormonal levels are normal. But what is normal? The normal range for T4 is from 4.5 to 11.5 ug/dl. In my practice I like to compare this range to that of shoe sizes which in the U.S. is numerically very similar. Are you a 5 or are you a 10? Don't try to fit me in a 10 shoe if I'm a 5! Any child can tell you that. In fact, according to your genes and specific medical history, your optimal thyroid levels could be anywhere in that wide range of what is considered normal! How then, do you know where your ideal level is? Because of this, finding the right dose of medication for each person can be time consuming since it requires a lot of trial and error with both you and your doctor keeping track of how you feel on different doses; but it is worth it for you to feel better.

Here's another way to look at this important concept. When a patient asks me, "What should my thyroid level be?" my response could be, "What should the thermostat in your house be set to?" The "normal" temperature in a person's home is a very individual choice. Forgetting the price of energy, the temperature should be set to what makes you most comfortable and that ideal comfort spot could be found anywhere within a wide range of "normal" temperatures. Now if you live with others, there may be a constant dispute about what the best temperature should be. If you work in my office you will see just how much thought goes into how and when to sneak up to change the thermostat (so annoying!!). So you see, there is no "should be" when it comes to thyroid levels, instead your optimal levels are the levels where you are most comfortable.

In addition, blood tests do not tell everything about hormone levels and their activity in the body. This is because, as we have seen, much of the T3 and T4 in the body is in an inactive form, and biologically active hormone is produced primarily in the target tissues. Therefore a blood test cannot by itself tell how much T3 or T4 there is in the cells where the hormone exerts its effects. This may also account for contradictory reports and misinformation (some even from doctors) about whether or not T3 treatments are effective. Research studies that do not ask the right questions may show for example, that T3 treatment is ineffective, or that changes in dosages do not have a significant effect.

Using Thyroid Function Tests To Diagnose Disease

Because there are many possible causes and presentations of hyperthyroidism and hypothyroidism, an accurate diagnosis and in-depth assessment of the cause of the disorder is necessary. A good starting place is to measure the TSH level in conjunction with T4 and T3 levels, plus the T3RU (T3 resin uptake) test, which allows the doctor to figure out how much of the hormone is actually "free." Remember it is only a tiny fraction of thyroid hormone that is not bound to blood proteins (therefore "free"), which is available to do the work. I have been asked by many of my patients to order free T4 and T3 levels. I find that commercial labs (where insurance companies send you for blood work) often don't do a very good job of performing these highly sensitive tests. So I compute the free hormone levels myself using the T3RU test.

Hyperthyroidism Treatments

There are several treatments for hyperthyroidism (an overactive thyroid):

- **Anti-thyroid drugs.** A class of drugs called suppressive thyrostatics, such as propylthiouracil (PTU) and methimazole (Tapazole), reduce the production of hormones by the thyroid. These drugs are by far doctors' favorites as the first line of treatment for hyperthyroidism. Both have been used with relative safety for 50 or more years. PTU has been the treatment of choice for pregnant and breast feeding women. Precautions for both drugs are required because side effects can occur though. Low white blood cell count leading to severe infection, abnormalities of liver function, generalized joint pains and itchy rash have all been reported. A very rare but potentially lethal form of liver failure has occurred with PTU, mostly in children. Neither I nor my colleagues in medical practice have ever seen or heard of a case though. In a move that surprised me, the FDA after 50 years of PTU being around, has just issued a strict warning about this complication, now leaving physicians to prescribe only Tapazole, except in rare situations.

- **Radioisotope therapy.** Commonly, radioactive iodine is given orally to reduce the thyroid's hormone production. The problem with this treatment is that radioactive iodine may cause the gland to temporarily or permanently shut down. This shut down can be treated with synthetic or natural thyroid hormone replacement. An overactive thyroid may eventually return to normal on its own though; an event called spontaneous remission. For that reason radioactive iodine treatment is generally reserved for those who after a year or so on medication treatment appear to be stuck with permanent hyperthyroidism.

- **Surgery.** This is an alternative to the above therapies, and involves removing a large section of the thyroid. Following surgery, thyroid hormone supplementation may be necessary to replace the thyroid hormones. Surgery is generally considered a last resort given the simplicity, safety and success of the other forms of treatment.

Hypothyroidism Treatments

Hypothyroidism (an underactive thyroid) is usually treated with prescription synthetic T4 hormone supplementation, Levothyroxine (known as Levothroid, Levoxyl, Synthroid, Unithroid and many others), either orally or injected. Dosage is particularly important and varies according to age, individual medical history, weight and diet. Treatment length varies, and is usually adjusted to eventually achieve "normal" TSH levels.

Oral doses of T3 (synthetic triiodothyronine) are sometimes added to T4-only treatment, depending on the professional philosophy of the physician. In general, the ATA and the American Association of Clinical Endocrinologists do not recommend the administration of T3 (because of potentially harmful side effects), but state that T4 supplementation is preferable because it allows the body to produce T3 naturally, via the body's regulatory system. Most doctors and endocrinologists endorse these practice guidelines, and prescribe T4-only treatments instead of the T3 plus T4 combination treatment. Here is a key point where I differ from the standards set by the AACE and other endocrine societies. More will be said about this below.

Within the Internet community there is a "buzz" about something called Wilson's Syndrome. According to the originator of this syndrome, Dr. Wilson, this syndrome results in low body temperature along with persistent symptoms of hypothyroidism. Dr. Wilson's preferred method of treatment of the syndrome is T3. I am unconvinced of the validity of Wilson's Syndrome and I am in agreement with the American Thyroid Association (ATA), which states there is no scientific support for the existence of Wilson's Syndrome.

T3 Plus T4 Combination Therapy

One of the most frustrating problems reported by members of Metabolism.com who have hypothyroidism is being unable to convince their doctor that treatment with Synthroid, Levoxyl or a similar synthetic T4 drug isn't working. The fact is that treatment with "T4-only" does not work for many patients, who remain plagued by their symptoms, including fatigue, weakness, the inability to concentrate or think clearly and the inability to lose weight. Very often, doctors view these patients as troublemakers, and continue to prescribe solely the T4 medication.

A recent discovery shows that genetic differences between individuals may be responsible for how effective T4 treatments are. Genetic differences in the amount of active T3 produced may explain why some patients need T3 treatment for hypothyroidism to restore normal functioning of their brain, muscles and heart, whereas others do not. Additionally, some people may also have difficulty converting T4 into T3 due to genetics.

In the Watts Study published in the *Journal of Clinical Endocrinology and Metabolism* in 2009, scientists investigated nearly 700 hypothyroid people, and found that a commonly inherited variation (polymorphism) in a gene was causing them not to respond to T4 medication, but to feel better with combination T3 and T4 therapy. Interestingly, this genetic difference does not affect blood thyroid hormone levels. That is because these people have less of the enzymes that convert T4 (the storage hormone) into T3 (the hormone that is more effective). Therefore, these people cannot effectively convert T4 into T3 inside their cells where it is needed, despite having T4 and T3 blood levels which are in the normal range. That is why they continue to not feel well on T4 therapy alone. Unfortunately, their blood test results are not able to tell doctors that they won't respond well to T4-only therapy.

People with this genetic variation (and perhaps other genetic variations that have yet to be discovered), comprise approximately 16% of the population. It is clear that these people will respond better to a combination therapy such as that provided by Armour Thyroid (because it contains both T3 and T4 in one pill) rather than taking drugs with T4 alone (like Synthroid). Alternately good results can also be seen with taking a T3 pill (like Cytomel) along with the Synthroid, although it is simpler to just take one Armour Thyroid pill to get both.

WARNING: Members at Metabolism.com have commented about purchasing thyroid hormone preparations via the Internet without a prescription. Others have referred to treating themselves with doses of T3. Thyroid hormones have very potent effects within the body. Please be aware you can seriously harm yourself or even die if the wrong amount of thyroid hormone is taken. DO NOT ATTEMPT TO TREAT YOURSELF WITH THYROID HORMONE. Thyroid treatment must be administered and supervised by a trained physician only.

The Bias Against Armour Thyroid

"Anyone know of an endocrinologist in Chicago who's open to combo therapy? I had this when I was pregnant and have never felt better. However, I can't find a doctor to do this now and am sick of leaving in tears knowing that this is the answer for ME, but no one cares enough to LISTEN and TRY."

Metabolism.com member

"Having a hard time finding someone in Charlotte, NC to work with me on medication other than Synthroid. Seems all that I've encountered are in this drug manufacturer's pocket. Any suggestions for this area?"

Metabolism.com member

"*The question I asked was, why so many physicians are refusing to prescribe T3 medications? I am an American lady, living in England for the last 17 years. I had medically intractable thyrotoxicosis, and a subsequent thyroidectomy. My surgery was 7 months ago, and I was put on Levothyroxine, 25 mcg, nocte, with a view to increasing the dosage to 75-100 mcg nocte. However, for some reason, I cannot tolerate any increase at all, and remained on 25. I felt terrible, my hair was falling out, and for the first time in my entire life I was gaining weight despite a 900 cal per day intake. My energy level was absolutely through the floor, and I was essentially bedridden, 8 days out of ten. I had come across Dr. Pepper's Metabolism. com site, and as a result, read up on T3 preparations, ie; Cytomel and Armour, which I believe is a T3/T4 combination drug. I took this information along to my surgeon, and he prescribed Liothyronine the same day. Now, the thing I cannot understand is, why the doctors in the US are not willing to do this. My surgeon had never prescribed Liothyronine for a patient, but I think that is because none of them had ever requested it. It has taken about 3 months, but I think I am finally beginning to feel some effect and benefit from the addition of the T3. I am really not able to find any reason for what almost appears to be a blanket refusal, among the U.S. physicians to prescribe it. Can ANYONE please explain this odd, and frankly incomprehensible impediment, to the recovery of at least some hypothyroid patients?? Input would most welcome.*"

Metabolism.com member

These Metabolism.com members are not isolated cases. There is significant mainstream clinical resistance to prescribing anything other than T4 alone, and Armour Thyroid in particular. I have a theory of how the bias against Armour thyroid and combination T4 plus T3 treatment evolved.

Armour Thyroid was among the earliest treatments for hypothyroidism. To create Armour, all the thyroid hormone in pig thyroid is extracted (as desiccated thyroid) and then concentrated or diluted to get to a standard dose per pill. All of the four thyroid hormone varieties are included in the compound, but by far the highest concentrations are that of T3 and T4 in a ratio of 20 to 80 (which is more T3 than found in the average human thyroid). It is important to remember the quoted ratio of T3 to T4 in the human thyroid, 7 to 93, is an average ratio and does not exclude the possibility of an individual having far different proportions.

Desiccated thyroid products were used for decades with great success and safety. Then, about 50 years ago, synthetic forms of thyroid hormone became available. Companies that manufactured synthetic thyroid hormone invested heavily in the thyroid research being performed by physician scientists at the major medical schools in the world. These physicians became the founders of the field of endocrinology and were the mentors of many generations of endocrinologists.

Scientists are, by definition, highly precise people. They are emotionally drawn to decimal points—the more the better. Synthetic thyroid hormone could be measured to the billionths of a gram and manipulated in a test tube and in the blood with incredible precision. Armour Thyroid is sloppy and crude by comparison. Eventually no one at the medical schools mentioned desiccated thyroid and that included combination T4 and T3 preparations as well. As a result, whole generations of endocrinologists/trainees have never heard of these products except as subjects of ridicule. How would I know this? Because that was the sort of training I received in the late 1970s and early 1980s.

As I have commented, physicians are generally reluctant to use a medication he or she has never used before, particularly one that has been derided by the leaders of the medical field. (For example, to my surprise, doctors at a recent meeting of the American Thyroid Association laughed openly at the idea of prescribing Armour Thyroid, even though some were in favor of combination T3 plus T4 therapy for patients who did not respond to T4 therapy alone.)

I was fortunate to have early exposure to the concept of combination T4 and T3 therapy through my contact with psychiatry research at Mt. Sinai. In the 1970s, research was showing the addition of T3 had a benefit with anti-depressant treatments so I developed an open mind about this approach. For many years thereafter, I gradually became more comfortable with combination therapy.

Even in the 1980s and 1990s when Armour Thyroid was being used by scammers with promises of weight loss and other unsubstantiated benefits, I saw the rationale for its use in the treatment of hypothyroidism. Little by little I incorporated it into my practice until the present when I enthusiastically prescribe it to those who have failed on T4-only treatment.

Other physicians trained in conventional settings remain mired in the principles taught by scientists whose careers were cut on Synthroid. For example, Dr. Thomas Repas wrote in the widely read *Endocrine Today* that he believed dried and powdered thyroid was old fashioned therapy and should no longer be used. What he was referring to was the fact that there used to be greater hormonal variation in Armour Thyroid than in synthetic hormones. Of course, the more recent techniques of concentrating or diluting to get a standard dose per pill eliminate that problem. However, his argument does not take into account that Armour Thyroid and similar treatments mimic the thyroid's natural production of T3 and T4 more closely than synthetic treatments do. Having never used these approaches how could endocrinologists like Dr. Repas be expected to embrace combination T4 plus T3 treatment or Armour Thyroid?

Interestingly, if you ask an endocrinologist scholar to show the studies demonstrating the clinical superiority of Synthroid to Armour Thyroid, I can tell you there aren't any or if any such studies exist, they would never pass as valid by modern standards. In my opinion, there are no scientific studies showing clinical superiority of synthetic thyroid hormone versus the desiccated variety. In my opinion, the overwhelming preponderance of synthetic T4 use by physicians in the U.S. in the treatment of thyroid disease is the result of outdated traditions without scientific support.

How to Talk to Your Endocrinologist

Based on the experiences reported by these and other members of Metabolism.com along with my personal experience meeting with other endocrinologists, I decided to prepare a script that could be used to get through to a doctor when requesting combination thyroid treatment. Doctors want to feel they are within the bounds of good science when prescribing a drug, particularly one that might be new to them. This is a good and wise thing. So with this new research in hand, hypothyroid individuals and their advocates can finally state with confidence that: "Yes! There is a firm scientific foundation for combination T4/T3 therapy. And, No! We are not just chronic complainers or kooks."

If I had hypothyroidism and was going to request a change in my thyroid treatment I would say something like, "Due to polymorphism (different varieties of a gene) of the deiodinase gene (the gene responsible for converting T4 into T3), I probably have a defective D2 deiodinase and therefore my peripheral conversion of T4 to T3 is impaired. I need T3 added to T4 to compensate for reduced intracellular T3 levels that cannot be detected on blood tests. Without T3, I continue to suffer with cellular hypothyroidism which is the likely cause of my persistent symptoms."

If you try this approach and your doctor looks bewildered hand them a copy of the Watts study in the *Journal of Clinical Endocrinology and Metabolism*, 2009, 94(5): 1623-1629. This can be downloaded from http://jcem.endojournals.org/content/94/5/1623.full.pdf+html and printed to take with you to your doctor's appointment.

The Recent Shortage of Armour Thyroid

As you realize, I preferentially prescribe Armour Thyroid, but there was a time not so long ago that it was no longer available. The sudden disappearance of Armour Thyroid from pharmacies in the United States in 2009 had all the makings of a mystery novel. Armour Thyroid had been available since the 1950s with a long history of being safe and effective. Then suddenly I was receiving numerous requests from pharmacies and prescription supply services requesting I rewrite my prescriptions of Armour due to lack of availability of certain pill strengths. For weeks I was able to get around this obstacle by utilizing the available Armour strengths in various combinations to arrive at the correct total dose. But eventually the Armour shortage became so severe that several locations said they were totally out of all Armour dosages and that an alternative treatment was required.

As anyone dealing with hypothyroidism would attest, it often takes many visits over many months to arrive at a satisfactory thyroid replacement plan. Once this finally happens, it's a relief to patients to know that their symptoms will be controlled by their specific medication plan. As a result, it can be very upsetting to have to change prescriptions if the medication is suddenly no longer available. Making matters worse, I was unable to explain why this shortage occurred and when, if ever, the medication would be available again.

Many of Metabolism.com members from all over the US were experiencing the same difficulties finding desiccated thyroid medications as well.

"WOW! I just called to have my prescription refilled, and I was shocked! Armour Thyroid has changed my life and I can't imagine going back to the foggy-thinking, exhausted way I was! I was so sick I had to stop working and I had asthma that couldn't be controlled. My children thought I was going to be sick and sleep forever…I CAN'T go back there! I tried synthetic thyroid products and I never responded, but Armour was like flipping a switch. I felt SO much better and now, because of money, the drug company is going to take wellness away from myself and so many others? This product is proven to work. Prescriptions are to make us well and to help us feel better. I certainly hope that the powers-that-be read what patients write here and take it to heart. HELP, PLEASE!"

Lori

"I don't know what I would do without Armour Thyroid. It gave me my life back when synthetic thyroid replacements couldn't. It's devastating to think about. Now I'm wondering how to fight back as my pharmacist carefully hands out small amounts of it as best as she can."

Laura

No one could produce a good reason for what was happening, not even the company, Forest Laboratories, that manufactured the drug. Several concerned Metabolism.com members contacted the FDA for clarification of the Armour situation and received a prepared statement in response:

> To date, there is not an approved drug application for the natural desiccated thyroid products. Without an approved drug application, the safety and efficacy has not been established by the FDA. Companies marketing natural desiccated thyroid products are encouraged to submit a new drug application (NDA) for approval.

> The Federal Food, Drug, and Cosmetic Act generally requires that drugs marketed in the United States be shown to be both safe and effective prior to marketing and widespread use in the general population. Drugs that are marketed without required FDA approval may not meet modern standards for safety, effectiveness, quality, and labeling.

> However, for a variety of historical reasons, some drugs, mostly older products, continue to be marketed illegally in the United States without required FDA approval. Many healthcare providers are unaware of the unapproved status of these drugs and have continued to unknowingly prescribe them because the drugs' labels do not disclose that they lack FDA approval. Often these drugs are advertised in reputable medical journals or are included in widely used pharmaceutical references such as the Physicians' Desk Reference (PDR)."

After studying this letter, I recognized key wording from the FDA that alerted me to potential political reasons for the Armour shortage. The explanation, as I saw it, was grounded in the fact that several thyroid medications such as Armour Thyroid (but also including synthetic T4 medications like Synthroid) existed before the FDA was given full regulatory power. In 1973 the Supreme Court empowered the FDA to regulate the use of prescription medications in the US. This meant that pharmaceutical companies would have to demonstrate, to the FDA's satisfaction, the safety and efficacy of all prescription drugs for specific indications before their use could be promoted. Medications like Synthroid and Armour, already vital components of medical therapy for years before 1973, entered a grey area of legitimacy after that time.

Just a few years ago, I was astounded to hear from my pharmaceutical representatives that Synthroid faced being banned by the FDA since it never provided the FDA with the type of documentation of safety and efficacy that all modern medications had. After 30 years the FDA decided it wanted to rescind the right of the drug manufacturer to promote this medication, which was considered safe and effective way before the FDA achieved regulatory power. What followed was a tense year during which the manufacturer of Synthroid went through the costly and bureaucratically intricate process needed for FDA approval, which it ultimately won.

Based on this information, I believed Armour Thyroid and other desiccated thyroid products were facing a similar situation. What convinced me of this is the wording in the FDA letter, which referred to Armour Thyroid as an "illegal drug." Basically, it seemed as though the FDA put Armour on its "Most Wanted List" and was intimidating the manufacturer (and prescribing physicians) by implying the law was being broken by continuing to make and use this drug.

In the case of Synthroid, which enjoys the full support by the medical community and provides millions of dollars in annual sales, the financial equation was a "no-brainer" in favor of putting the money into the process to gain approval. Not so for Armour Thyroid, which had been defamed by the American Academy of Clinical Endocrinologists (AACE) and whose use was much more limited and far less profitable to the manufacturer. I speculated that the pharmaceutical company had already done the math and decided that not making Armour makes more financial sense than to continue making the "illegal" product and going through the FDA gauntlet for approval.

Later I got confirmation that political and economic, not medical, forces were responsible for Armour Thyroid's sudden disappearance in the form of a letter from the President and Chief Operating Officer of Forest Labs, Lawrence Olanoff, M.D, Ph.D. This letter revealed that Forest Labs entered into an agreement with the federal government to accept fines and other penalties in a settlement of misdemeanor and felony charges related to the company's marketing practices of its Celexa and Levothroid products.

It was clear to me that in the midst of negotiations with the FDA on these issues, Forest Labs needed to be ultra-cautious in its handling of Armour Thyroid, which was separately being scrutinized by the FDA for formulation issues. Was it a coincidence back then that Medicare removed Armour from its list of recognized drugs or was it a warning by the government that Armour was on the "hit" list? The executives at Forest undoubtedly were required to remain silent as they dealt with the government on these issues.

The good news is that the Armour shortage is over, coinciding with the settlement between Forest and the FDA. It was a difficult time for many people who needed Armour and for the doctors who depended on it for adequate treatment of hypothyroidism. But, if I am correct, this should be the end of this painful episode.

CHAPTER 6

Diabetes Treatment

There are an estimated 16 million diabetics in the United States today. This number can be further subdivided into type 1 (juvenile-onset) or type 2 (adult-onset) diabetics. At the root of both types of diabetes is the inability to control levels of blood glucose, the main energy source for the human body. This is due to either a deficiency or developed insensitivity to insulin, which controls the uptake of glucose from the bloodstream into the cells.

There are many long-term complications that can accompany diabetes, including stroke, heart disease, kidney disease, blindness, and loss of sensation in the limbs, all due to an excess of glucose in the blood. As a result $1 in every $10 spent on healthcare in the US is spent trying to control blood sugar levels, delay the onset of the disease and slow the progression of diabetes complications. But there is good news and bad news when it comes to current diabetes care. Let's start with the bad news first.

The Bad News—Major Stumbles in the Treatment of Diabetes

Stumbles and false starts have marred the treatment of diabetes in the US for the past few years, with many of them coming from the supposed "expert" bodies that direct care in this country.

The Call for Tight Glycemic Control

For several years the leaders of the endocrine community, including the American Academy of Endocrinologists (AACE), have been promoting stricter guidelines for maintaining near normal blood sugar levels in diabetics, particularly for those who are in the hospital. For hospitalized diabetics, tight control means keeping their blood sugar in the normal "non-diabetic" range 24 hours a day, seven days a week. For diabetics not in the hospital, the goal is a glycohemoglobin A1c level of less than 6%, which is considered the dividing line between diabetic and normal blood sugars.

The science behind the call for this degree of blood sugar control for diabetics, particularly for hospitalized patients, is flimsy at best. It is based on just a few small studies with questionable study design and defies the common knowledge that it takes more than 10 years to see physical evidence of high blood sugar on body organs. In addition, clinicians with years of experience treating diabetes in hospitalized patients have seen that non-ideal blood sugar levels rarely have any clinical impact on their patients' outcomes.

Even more telling is that recent major studies have proven that not only does this rigorous degree of tight control not benefit hospitalized and non-hospitalized diabetics, but also that the death and complication rates were even higher for tightly controlled patients. Most notably, the NIH (National Institutes of Health) recently called for the ACCORD study to end. This is a study that examined the response of tight glycemic control on outpatient diabetics with a high risk for heart disease and stroke. The ACCORD study was ended early when it became clear that "tight" glycemic control resulted in worse outcomes for diabetics than conventional glucose control!

As far as studies of diabetics in the intensive care unit, back as far as 2003, a UK study revealed worse outcomes with tight control. Hopefully putting an end to the quest for this seemingly ill-conceived goal are the results of the NICE-SUGAR study recently published in the *New England Journal of Medicine* showing increased death rates for diabetics receiving tight glycemic control in the intensive care unit.

Making matters worse, this dangerously aggressive approach adds substantially to the cost and nursing requirements. For hospitalized diabetic patients with an enormous range of illnesses, stresses, diets and requirements for diagnostic procedures, instituting tight blood sugar control requires a special nurse for each patient and creates a logistical nightmare for the hospital.

2010 Diabetes Treatment Guidelines Lack Credibility

In 2010, the American Academy of Clinical Endocrinologists (AACE) issued new treatment guidelines for the treatment of type 2 diabetes. Complex medical guidelines are often referred to as a treatment algorithm. One of the stated goals of the AACE algorithm is to focus primarily on the theoretical ability of the diabetic medications to control blood sugar, while ignoring the cost of the medication. The rationale to this approach is that controlling blood sugar with more expensive drugs will cost less in the long run since patients will be healthier and have fewer complications due to better control of their blood sugar. On the surface this philosophy seems sound but digging beneath the surface reveals dangerous flaws in this thinking.

1. The first assumption, that newer medications for diabetes are better than older drugs, is unsubstantiated. In fact there is ample evidence that newer diabetic drugs are sometimes worse than the older drugs for controlling blood sugar levels. The latest study finding no benefit of the newer diabetes medications is the FIELD study conducted outside of the US. This study showed that 5 years of treatment with older diabetic drugs, like sulfonylureas, metformin and insulin, resulted in adequate and prolonged control of blood sugar. In 2007 researchers from Johns Hopkins Bloomberg School of Public Health summarized the results of major studies using older and newer anti-diabetic medications and found no significant benefit of the newer medications.

2. The next assumption, that cost is not a key factor in treatment success, contradicts most clinicians' experience in diabetes care. It is clear to me that patients are far less likely to comply with using expensive drugs than medications they can more easily afford. Looking at the numbers reveals the vast cost differences between the older (generic) versus the newer (brand name) medications. Using figures provided by a local pharmacy I found that the retail cost of a typical two-drug therapy for diabetes using older drugs was $59 per month. The retail cost of using two of the new drugs for a month ranged from $481 to $570. In more severe cases of diabetes, three drugs per day may be needed. With three drugs, the low cost alternative amounts to $185 per month while the high-end alternative with new drugs is $610 per month.

Looking at the cost of using insulin shows a similar vast cost difference between the older and newer drugs. Older forms of insulin may cost $100 for a month's supply while a similar course of therapy with the newer insulin preparations will cost almost $250 per month. How many people will be willing and able to afford the new versus the old drugs, particularly knowing that there may be no health benefit to the more expensive drug combination?

The end result of not being able to afford these prices is non-compliance with medications, and the result of non-compliance is higher costs passed on to the medical system. The Medco study from 2005 showed that the least compliant patients were more than twice as likely to be hospitalized compared to the most compliant, and that the yearly cost of caring for non-compliant patients is double that of compliant patients.

3. My next point is possibly the most controversial. The AACE guidelines were produced by a committee of highly respected and qualified physicians. However many are also highly compensated consultants to the pharmaceutical companies that market the newest generation of diabetes medications. In the disclaimer attached to the committee's recommendations, committee members revealed consulting arrangements with virtually every one of the pharmaceutical companies whose interests are affected by their committee's findings.

I too am a consultant to many of these same companies (at least until now), but I am not responsible for developing national guidelines for diabetes care. In my opinion the close association of the committee to pharmaceutical companies takes away from the credibility of their recommendations. The need for credibility is even more important when the AACE committee advises physicians to avoid using sulfonylureas. This is the only class of drugs not marketed by any of the big pharma companies and also happens to be the cheapest drug class, the drugs with the longest history of use, and the class of drugs many regard as the most effective at lowering blood sugar levels. The sulfonylurea class of drugs is so effective at lowering blood sugar that they are used as the gold standard by which the effectiveness of all new diabetic medications are compared.

Here is a clear example of how these treatment guidelines (as well as big pharma) have failed to protect the needs of diabetics who may already be disadvantaged by financial circumstances and disease. This is the story of one of my patients, an elderly, blind and impoverished woman with blindness due to diabetes. She managed to maintain some degree of independence and did not complain about what a lousy hand life had dealt her. One of the ways she remained independent was by using a device known as an insulin pen. The pen is an all-in-one device equipped with a needle that contains an insulin reservoir and is adjusted to a specific insulin dose by a twist of its dial. With this device she was able to inject her insulin dose daily by herself with sufficient accuracy to control her diabetes. The older method of using a separate syringe and insulin vial required too much dexterity and vision for her to use safely and would have required someone to help her on a regular basis.

The type of insulin she used, NPH, dissolved slowly so her risk of low blood sugar (hypoglycemia) was less than if she used the newer insulins containing rapid-acting insulin. What's more, NPH insulin was still relatively inexpensive, costing about one half the price of the newer insulins.

At one of her visits to my office, I learned her NPH insulin pen was being discontinued and there was nothing on the market to replace it. The only insulin pens that were available contained insulin with rapid action or were at least twice as expensive as her present pen.

What could have caused this sudden shift in the medical supply chain? The answer was the American Association of Clinical Endocrinologists (AACE) new Diabetic Treatment Guidelines, which dismissed NPH insulin as outdated and recommended the newer (more expensive) insulins be used in its place. The company's decision to stop making NPH insulin pens coincided almost simultaneously with this new AACE policy statement.

Diabetes is the most common cause of blindness in the U.S. My guess is that there are more blind, poor diabetics who could make good use of the inexpensive NPH insulin pen. In the case of my patient, we scrambled to put together a support plan for her so she can maintain her independence, her pocket book and still control her diabetes to a reasonable degree. However, I'm sure there were some patients who were not so lucky.

> NEWS FLASH: At the time of putting this book together, Eli Lilly and Company has an NPH pen available. This pen costs $150 per 1000 units of insulin. At Walmart a 1000 unit vial of the same insulin costs $25. The pen, costing 6 times as much as a vial, is not really a bargain but if you're blind and desperate, you might just be willing to pay the difference.

Setbacks in Diabetes Drug Development

In 2007 an alarm was sounded by several outspoken critics whose analysis pointed to an increased cardiovascular risk associated with Avandia use. This is one of only two available medicines with unique properties to treat diabetes and was approved in 1999. Several years later, research studies seemed to indicate a small increased risk of heart attacks in people who used Avandia. Ever since then, there has been a heated debate over whether this was a true risk or just the result of overly aggressive interpretation of the available data.

There are two major analyses on the subject of heart attack risk with Avandia. One, written by a doctor on the payroll of a competing drug company, looked at results from 14,000 patients taking Avandia and found a small increased risk of heart attack or stroke. The other study analyzed another 14,000 Avandia users and found no such association.

To gain a better understanding of the true Avandia risk, I went back to the actual data submitted by Dr. Nissan and colleagues in the study that reviewed all the available clinical data on Avandia. This was the study that ignited this controversy (the first study mentioned above). What I found supports my notion that the real risk is doctors and researchers manipulating statistics to show whatever they want it to show.

In Dr. Nissan's review of 42 studies that compared Avandia to other diabetes treatments, results from a total of 27,843 diabetics were analyzed (15,560 received Avandia and 12,283 took other treatments).

During the study period there were a total of 158 heart attacks and 58 deaths from cardiovascular causes. Compared to the other treatments, there were 14 extra heart attacks in the Avandia group. If your first reaction is "whoa! 14 extra deaths seems unacceptable," remember that there were 2,300 more people in the Avandia group for bad things to happen to.

The overall occurrence of cardiovascular death for diabetics in the US is generally accepted as 65% or more, and the occurrence of heart attacks is substantially higher. In Nissan's study of 27,843 total diabetics, 65% is equal to 17,730 total heart attacks. The 14 extra heart attacks in the Avandia group would make the heart attack rate 65.09%. Not a very alarming increase if it were true. In the other treatments group, if we accounted for the smaller number of participants in that group, we would find that the heart attack occurrence would be higher at 65.12% (72 heart attacks with Avandia and 91 heart attacks with other treatments, if you are interested in the math).

This means that the "higher than average" number of heart attacks with Avandia occurs once per every 1250 patients. For practitioners who treat diabetes and understand the enormous degree of variation between diabetic patients, trying to pinpoint the factors accounting for one heart attack per 1250 in this group would be like trying to isolate one snowflake in a blizzard. I simply do not believe that there is a way to validate the results of Dr. Nissan's study. Believing that statistics can correctly pinpoint the cause of 1 in 1250 heart attacks within the chaos that is diabetes care, in my opinion, is being naïve to the true complexity of this disease and its treatment. Plus, remember that the other treatments caused approximately 1.5 heart attacks per every 1250 patients!

Still, most people do not share my opinion, and on May 18, 2011, the FDA announced new restrictions on the prescribing, dispensing and use of Avandia and other rosiglitazone-containing medications like Avandamet and Avandaryl. The FDA also stated that after November 18, 2011, these medications will not be available through retail pharmacies. This essentially ends the use of Avandia to treat diabetes in the US and other countries.

According to the FDA, this decision was based on studies showing that Avandia triggers more heart attacks than its competitor, Actos. However, Actos hasn't fared much better in recent years when it comes to safety trials. Actos had been withdrawn in France due to concerns that it may cause bladder cancer but has recently been reinstated since the scientific evidence for the cancer connection was not found to be substantiated (so far). As of yet it hasn't been withdrawn in the US although the FDA did issue a warning that individuals with bladder cancer or at risk for bladder cancer should be advised not to use Actos. This is a sure sign of trouble, and if Actos is hit hard by these actions this whole class of diabetes drugs (thiazolidinediones) may be eliminated from use.

But this isn't the only fall-out from the entire Avandia/Actos debacle. The FDA has been widely criticized for allowing this supposed public danger to go unrecognized for so long. Many think that it is in response to this criticism that the FDA was forced to add new, much more stringent requirements to the approval process for new drugs.

Some pharmaceutical executives believe the new FDA requirements will double the cost of bringing a new drug to market. Approval of several promising new diabetes treatments has already been stalled and the companies developing new medical therapies are beginning to move diabetes treatments to the backburner.

For example, two new medications with potential use in diabetic treatment failed in their attempts to reach the U.S. market. Galvus (marketed by Novartis) was set to become one of the first of a new type of medication for lowering elevated blood sugar in diabetes, but it was denied approval by the FDA due to safety concerns. The FDA also rejected another promising drug, Ramonabant (a weight loss drug shown to improve various metabolic problems in diabetics) over safety issues.

Safety has become such a huge issue with the FDA and doctors alike partially as a result of medical opportunism. It is impossible to ignore the lawyer ads on TV that start with; "Have you or your loved ones been injured by (fill in the blank)?! Then you may be entitled to substantial financial compensation." Endocrinologists have been seeing more of the prescription drugs they prescribe in these ads than any other specialty, and it would be naïve to think this type of negative publicity is lost on physicians.

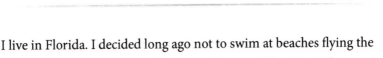

I live in Florida. I decided long ago not to swim at beaches flying the red flag warning of shark sightings in the area. Likewise, I shy away from prescribing medications that the lawyers are circling, even if I otherwise regard the medication as safe and effective. This is exactly what's happening with Avandia and Actos.

Lawsuits against Avandia have been underway for some time and Actos appears to be next on the hit list. Some people may make money in this process but unfortunately, everyone else will wind up a loser, and here's why.

The lawsuits against Avandia will contend that the medication caused heart attack or stroke. The truth of this contention is very much in question (as I explained earlier), but the murkiness of the water doesn't stop the lawyers from trying to take a bite out of the flesh of GSK (GlaxoSmithKline), the maker of Avandia.

Undeterred by the lack of conclusive data the opportunists have plunged in for the quick buck. Advertisements fill my email in-box from lawyers looking for customers who want to sue the drug manufacturer in class action lawsuits. Try Googling "Avandia side effects" and you will find the first several pages of results are ads looking for lawsuit clients.

In the last month alone I've received two requests for patient records from these lawyers. Both patients had heart disease at the time they started the medication. One patient who recently died was over 80 years old, and the other, who had significant heart disease and other diabetes complication to begin with, is still alive more than 7 years after treatment with Avandia. I wonder how much benefit these patients received from the medication allowing them to survive as long as they did despite all the problems they had related to their diabetes.

Why should you care about whether a small army of opportunists who each get a few thousand dollars from the drug manufacturer and a handful of lawyers who have become millionaires? Because it is just this sort of legal action which is convincing drug makers to back away from developing other potential diabetes treatments. It takes a decade and a billion dollars to bring a new drug in front of the FDA. This doesn't include the cost of developing drugs that fail to even make it to FDA review. Then the FDA approval process is tortuous and uncertain. Passing this hurdle, any new drug can come under attack (like Avandia) for "possible" side effects, making the company vulnerable to devastating legal costs and bad publicity.

It just isn't economically feasible to develop new diabetes drugs in the United States any more. As a result, new drug development is grinding to a halt. And unfortunately we will all suffer due to lack of innovation, not only for diabetes treatment but also for the treatment of many other dangerous diseases.

The Failure of Inhaled Insulin

The FDA approved the first inhaled insulin, known as Exubera, in January 2006. However, by October 2007, Pfizer (the pharmaceutical giant with sole rights for marketing the drug) announced it had decided to end its role in selling this drug. This announcement effectively ended the availability of Exubera in the US, and patients taking this medication were faced with being switched to something else.

The reason for Pfizer's abandonment of Exubera appeared to be slow sales due to the lack of interest by consumers in using inhaled insulin. Physicians were also slow to recommend this treatment due to the difficulties in teaching patients how to use the inhaler device and restrictions on using inhaled insulin in patients with minor lung disorders.

Despite the failure of Exubera, other versions of the drug and inhalers were still being developed by various pharma companies. Unfortunately, Exubera was later linked to the development of lung cancer, effectively ending any chance that Exubera (or any other inhaled insulin) could return to the market even if the delivery problems were solved.

Dangerous Commercial Weight Loss Programs

Ads on TV and in magazines are promoting weight loss programs specifically designed for diabetics. While weight loss is crucial to successful treatment of type 2 diabetes and is a highly desirable goal, in practice it can be dangerous if not properly supervised.

Many adult diabetics are taking powerful medications to lower their blood sugar since they are unable to maintain good glucose control with diet and exercise alone. These medications can work through several different mechanisms in the body, some of which can lead to hypoglycemia (dangerously low blood sugar). Hypoglycemia may occur almost without warning, resulting in a rapid heartbeat, sweating, confusion, poor coordination and even unconsciousness. When a diabetic begins a weight loss program, if their medication is not adjusted appropriately the risk of hypoglycemia goes up dramatically. I've seen evidence of this in my office.

A few months ago, I was concluding a visit with a patient with thyroid disease, while her diabetic husband, who was also my patient, looked on. They are a pleasant older couple I have known for years, and they are devoted to helping each other stay healthy. As they were leaving the exam room, the wife apologetically turned the subject to her husband mentioning he was having almost daily "episodes" of weakness and confusion.

"I hadn't changed his diabetic medication recently so why should his blood sugar be a problem now?" I thought. A number of other unpleasant possibilities immediately occurred to me. I inquired about signs of a possible stroke or heart condition. If these other angles were unproductive I faced the choice of sending him to the hospital for an evaluation. We quickly ran through a routine review of his symptoms. He had lost 10 pounds in the past month, the wife mentioned. "Oh no! cancer," was my first thought. His wife explained that as a New Year's resolution he enrolled in a commercial weight loss program for diabetics. With relief, I knew we had the explanation of his disturbing new symptoms—hypoglycemia.

But what if they hadn't come in to see me that day? What if this man's symptoms continued? Imagine if his symptoms suddenly occurred when he was behind the wheel. The potentially disastrous results are all too common down here in Florida. I am just thankful that my patient's wife stopped and mentioned her husband's new symptoms at the last moment that day because a far worse outcome for her husband was possible.

Although most of the weight loss programs being advertised are designed by professionals, they are being administered by people without any medical background. And unfortunately, despite having overall good intentions, it seems to me that these programs are putting people at risk and are equivalent to engaging in practicing medicine without a license. It is careless to assume that the dieter's doctor will be in a position to immediately make accurate medication adjustments when the diet begins. The result, as with my patient, is the development of potentially serious complications of hypoglycemia.

Perhaps the Biggest Stumble of Them All

Finally, in what could rank as one of the longest stumbles in medical history, in 2008 the American Diabetes Association finally gave its support to a low carbohydrate diet as a method for weight loss in diabetics. This occurred a mere 26 years after Dr. Robert Atkins published his world famous low carbohydrate weight loss method!

The Good News—What Really Works

In working with diabetes patients in my practice I have found that the people who are the most successful in managing their condition are those who are the most motivated to take good care of themselves. There are so many people who think with all of the medications like insulin and the different pills available that if they just take their medication they'll be okay. And that's just not true. You really need to know the right things to eat, avoid unhealthy habits and exercise regularly to do well at controlling your diabetes.

Diet and Exercise

Type 2 diabetes, or adult onset diabetes, is generally seen in overweight adults. When an individual gains weight, the body must produce more and more insulin to compensate for the additional fat. Once the pancreas has reached maximum insulin production, it cannot produce enough insulin to keep the blood sugar normal. The result is called type 2 diabetes.

Unfortunately losing weight to control diabetes isn't as simple as it sounds.

> "It can be difficult to even know where to begin when embarking on a weight loss program to shed those extra pounds especially when nothing else seems to have worked."
>
> **Moises**

If you are truly going to make a change that will bring your glucose under control and help you lose weight, you will have to take control of what you and your family eat. It is less difficult than you think. The secret is in your commitment to change. Here are some specific hints to help you make good food choices while you are shopping:

- Prepare ahead. We've all run out for a few things and ended up buying twice as much as we needed. Often, something in the store tempts us to do just that. For example, many supermarkets position the bakery right where you walk in, with the wonderful smell of newly baked bread or cakes perfuming the air. It's not an accident.

- Consult your cookbooks and create a weekly menu. Write down all of the ingredients you need for it.

- Know what you are going to make, and make sure that most of what you buy fits into your overall meal plan.

- Check the fridge and pantry so you know what you don't need to buy.

- Shop weekly. Shopping too often or stretching your shopping trips to every two weeks will make sticking to your meal plan more difficult.

- Learn the store layout. The fewer tempting products you see and the less time you spend browsing, the easier it will be to avoid buying the wrong foods. The healthiest fresh foods are in areas against the store walls. Don't spend time in the central aisles with things you don't need.

- Look up and down. The most attractively packaged food is on shelves at eye level. Healthy foods tend to be higher or lower.

- Stay away from the areas where store employees are offering free samples of high-carb, fatty foods.

- Eat before you shop. A hungry shopper buys more food and makes worse food choices, plus with diabetes, you need to eat at specific times and in amounts that ensure stable blood sugar.

- Shop alone, without the kids. Although research claims that men are more likely to stick to their list only, the levels of obesity in both genders suggest otherwise. Going to the supermarket should be a directed, time-limited event. You are there to buy certain things you need; you don't have to review every single one of the store's offerings. If possible, shop for food when the kids are in school because they are special targets for marketers.

- Make healthy choices. This doesn't only mean buying fresh vegetables from local farms or good produce in the supermarket. A healthy choice is a meal you make at home rather than take-out or prepared foods. Over the past decade, sales of prepared foods at the deli counters and throughout the store have risen steadily.

Americans now spend over $15 billion per year on prepared foods in supermarkets and in shopping mall food courts.

- Ask questions. You'd be surprised how much help the people behind the counters can be and not only at high-end supermarkets.

- While sales of starchy, fat-dripping fast foods are dropping, prepared take-out foods aren't much better. The choices are often "family friendly": fried chicken, chicken nuggets, chicken wings, baked potatoes, egg rolls, tacos, and creamy "comfort food" soups. Did you know that much of the prepared supermarket foods are made by the same giant food companies that make fast foods? If you buy prepared foods, avoid those with heavy mayonnaise or breading and high calories. Dodge items featuring rice or mashed potatoes, as well.

- Some experts suggest you take a close look at how much of your diet comes from the prepared choices. If prepared food makes up more than half of your diet, you have a problem. While one solution would be to cook more or learn to cook better, some people simply don't like to cook or have too little time to make meals at home. But this isn't an insurmountable problem. It just takes some scheduling and/or some cooking lessons.

Weight Loss Surgery

Diet and exercise are not the only ways to improve your weight and your diabetes. On-going research continues to confirm that weight loss surgery can improve and even reverse type 2 diabetes. A recent study conducted at NYU Medical Center recruited approximately 100 people with type 2 diabetes to undergo gastric banding. The results showed that almost half of the participants returned to normal glucose levels following the surgery without needing anti-diabetic medication, while the other half were able to significantly reduce the amount of medication they needed to control their diabetes. In addition to this dramatic reduction in their medication requirement, these diabetics had substantial weight loss.

The rapid weight loss promoted by gastric by-pass or gastric banding surgery causes the body to decline in size to a point where the pancreas is once again able to supply the proper amounts of insulin and the diabetes is "cured". However, if the person regains the weight, the diabetes will return. Some experts believe that gastric surgery also improves other hormones that affect blood sugar and that the weight loss itself is not the key to seeing better blood sugar levels. Either way, it works.

Weight loss surgery is not like cosmetic surgery, though. The risks are seen as relatively greater than cosmetic surgery, and there are frequent complications involving the digestive system. Costs of surgery are high and are generally not covered by insurance. That's why many people travel outside of the US to have the surgery at a lower cost.

Currently in the US, the guideline for consideration for surgical treatment of diabetes is a BMI (body mass index) of greater than 40 or a BMI of 35 or more associated with some complication of diabetes such as leg ulceration. Doctors are now struggling to decide if these guidelines should be relaxed so more people with diabetes would qualify for weight loss surgery.

Incretins

For the last 6 years a new class of drugs have been available for diabetes treatment—they are based on chemicals known as incretins. Incretins are natural hormones released from specialized cells in the small intestine into the bloodstream after a meal. These hormones stimulate the pancreas to produce insulin so that rising blood glucose levels can be brought down.

While there isn't just one type of incretin, the most important for people with diabetes is called glucagon-like peptide-1 (GLP-1). Research has shown that people with type 2 diabetes don't produce enough GLP-1, which may be the underlying reason why they can't control high blood glucose levels.

GLP-1 has more responsibilities in the body than simply stepping up insulin production after a meal though. Because of its actions in the body, GLP-1 also reduces appetite and helps with weight loss. It may also improve heart health by lowering cholesterol and triglyceride levels in the blood—all very good things for people with diabetes.

METABOLISM.com

So why can't people with diabetes just take GLP-1 and be done with it? After all, doctors prescribe insulin to boost or replace natural insulin production all the time. It turns out that supplementing GLP-1 levels isn't that easy. In the body, as soon as an incretin like GLP-1 is made, a special enzyme (called DPP-4) is on its trail. Just like a tiny Pac-Man, this enzyme chases GLP-1 down and chomps it to bits. This quickly reduces GLP-1 levels in the body until another meal causes more to be produced. While this process is essential to regulating normal metabolism, for people with diabetes who already have low GLP-1 levels, getting around this enzyme is essential for treatment.

To combat this problem, researchers started searching for chemicals that looked and acted like incretins in the body but were not broken down by the DPP-4 enzyme. One of the first was discovered in the 1990s in a type of lizard (Gila monster) venom. The resulting drug that was based on this discovery, exenatide (brand name Byetta), was approved in 2005.

Because exenatide and other incretin-like drugs are made out of protein, they need to be injected and cannot be taken as pills because they would be digested in the stomach. Still, exanatide only has about an eight-hour life span in the body and must be taken twice a day around mealtimes. Another similar drug, Victoza, sticks around in the body for longer but it still needs to be administrated every day.

Researchers have found that the longer incretin-based drugs remain active in the body, the better. For that reason, Amylin Pharmaceuticals, the makers of Byetta (exanatide), are working on a version that would only need to be taken once a week. This new drug, known by the brand name Bydureon, is set to be approved by the FDA in early 2012, which may mark a true advance in diabetes care, if people can afford it.

CHAPTER 7

Hormone Treatments

As morbid and depressing as it may sound, every stage our body goes through from the moment we are born takes us one step closer to our inevitable death. After birth, most living things are programmed to develop physically and sexually, to rise to dominance in their environment, pass on their genetic material as fast and as frequently as they can, and then they die. And what is the thing calling the shots, transitioning the body from one of these programmed stages of life onto the next? That's right—hormones.

During the development years (up to age 25 or so) the natural suicide genes programmed into our cells (known as apoptosis genes) mostly serve constructive purposes like removing tissues that stand in the way of growth or preventing cancer cells from reproducing. The chemical messages of growth and development produced in our endocrine glands (known as hormones) are released into our blood in abundant amounts. These hormones include growth hormone, sex hormones like testosterone and estrogen, and adrenal hormones such as DHEA. After that these hormones gradually decrease and our abilities and physical attributes begin to decline.

The onset of menopause is the most obvious example of a natural ending of the hormone-making process. The estrogen deficiency caused by menopause induces changes in the skin, hair, bone and arteries (arthrosclerosis), not to mention hot flashes, moodiness and a loss of libido that reduces quality of life. Less obvious but just as significant hormonal declines associated with aging, are the steady dwindling of testosterone in men and the reduction of growth hormone and DHEA levels in both sexes. Because of the negative impacts that dwindling amounts of these care-taking hormones can have on the body, the question is whether or not replacement of these hormones can delay aging and/or improve the quality of our lives.

> IMPORTANT NOTICE: Hormones such as growth hormone, testosterone and DHEA are prescription drugs that must be prescribed by a licensed professional within a doctor-patient relationship. Prescribing or using growth hormone for the purpose of enhancing athletic performance or using these hormones without a prescription is illegal and punishable by fines and possible jail time.

Hormone Replacement Therapy—Estrogen

According to the North American Menopause Society, every year millions of menopausal women between the ages of 30 to 60 go to their doctors in search of relief from hot flashes, night sweats, bloating, headaches, insomnia, fatigue, mood swings, depression, weight gain, anxiety attacks, aging skin, irritability, foggy thinking and bone loss. For decades, the most common solution for the miseries of menopause was hormone replacement therapy (HRT) with estrogen. However, it was abandoned almost overnight in 2002 when researchers at the National Institutes of Health (NIH) abruptly ended a major clinical trial of the risks and benefits of combined HRT in women known as the Women's Health Initiative (WHI). After more than five years of using a combination estrogen-progestin drug, the women showed an increase in the risk of breast cancer, stroke, blood clots and heart attacks. This announcement caused thousands of women to contact their doctors to see if they should continue their treatment or find alternative therapies. So is taking HRT really a big mistake?

Heart Health

Women have a much lower risk of heart attacks then men until they reach menopause. At menopause when the ovaries stop making estrogen the risk of having a heart attack climbs rapidly until it equals that of men. Common sense suggests that if losing estrogen causes increased heart risks then replacing estrogen should prevent them. What the WHI appears to show is that HRT does not protect women from heart attacks and instead may actually increase their risk more than menopause alone does. Part of this increased risk may be linked to the issue of blood clots associated with estrogen treatment. This is likely due to the effect of estrogen in increasing certain blood proteins that promote the development of blood clots.

However, in 2008, a Danish study countered these results. This study, which was the largest to look at the effects of HRT since the WHI trial was stopped early, found that there was no overall increase in the risk of heart attacks in women who used HRT compared to women who had never taken it. It did find, though, there was a risk for younger women. Women between the ages of 51 and 54 who were taking HRT during the study had a 24% greater risk of heart attacks than women who had never taken HRT.

The study also found that the type of HRT and the way the women took it made a huge difference in the risk of heart attacks. Taking a continuous combination of estrogen and progesterone increased heart attack risk by 35%, while taking HRT on a cyclical basis (estrogen followed by a combination of estrogen and progesterone) tended to lead to a reduced risk of heart attacks. These results suggest that taking HRT in cycles may be a better option.

To deal with the risks associated with increased blood clotting with estrogen, my thought is that adding a simple baby aspirin daily may be the answer just as baby aspirin is now recommended for those at increased risk of heart attack. Unfortunately, aspirin is unlikely to be helpful in preventing blood clots referred to as DVT, which occur in veins (usually in the legs), but this is not known for sure. As with all medications, there are downsides to aspirin such as gastric irritation and ulcer bleeding, but these risks can be assessed by the individual and their doctor.

Breast Cancer

Probably the biggest cause for concern regarding post-menopausal HRT highlighted by the WHI study was an increased risk of breast cancer. This finding applied to women in the WHI who were using combination estrogen and progesterone replacement. Progesterone is given to reduce the risk of estrogen causing uterine (endometrial) cancer, but it is not crucial for relief of post-menopausal symptoms. Interestingly, women who used estrogen replacement alone (without the progesterone) actually showed no increase and possibly even a reduction in invasive breast cancer after 7 years on the treatment. In the group of women who started "estrogen only" replacement more than 5 years after entering menopause, the reduction in breast cancer was even bigger. Experts therefore conclude that "estrogen only" HRT is likely to be considerably safer from a breast cancer point of view, and starting estrogen five years after menopause reduces the cancer risk even further.

A new class of drugs, known as SERMs, have shown promising results in clinical studies when used in combination with estrogen. SERMs, like the drug Evista, help protect against the uterine-cancer-causing effect of estrogen, so progesterone is no longer needed with HRT. This immediately reduces many of the undesirable effects of HRT found in the WHI study, including lowering breast cancer risk and cholesterol levels. This combination of drugs is referred to as a tissue-selective estrogen complex (TSEC).

Other advantages of TSEC treatment are improvements in bone density (lower osteoporosis risk) and possible reduction in the development of coronary artery disease. Although TSEC treatment is not yet FDA approved for treatment of post-menopausal symptoms, individual doctors can prescribe this if they feel the available information is favorable and the risk/benefit ratio is in favor of the patient's well being.

The relationship between HRT and breast cancer risk is further complicated by the finding that post-menopausal women using HRT who develop breast cancer appear to have better survival and less aggressive tumors than post-menopausal women who are diagnosed with breast cancer and never used HRT. Breast cancer may not be caused by estrogen, but cancer may grow more rapidly in the presence of estrogen. This doesn't sound like an advantage but small, undetected cancers may grow rapidly with HRT so that they can be seen on a mammogram and be removed in their early stages before they have the chance to spread.

Benefits of Estrogen: Brain Function and Blood Pressure

Despite these risks, estrogen therapy still provides women with very real benefits. A recently published study in the journal *Neurology* shows that women who undergo premature menopause due to surgical removal of one or both ovaries and who don't receive estrogen replacement, have a significantly higher risk of developing memory loss, dementia (senility) and Parkinson's Disease in later years. This means that the younger the women were at the time of menopause, the greater their risk of having brain dysfunction later in life.

While this study didn't investigate why this happened, another group of researchers may have found the answer. Researchers gave post-menopausal women one dose of inhaled estrogen while measuring blood flow to their brain. They discovered that the estrogen caused an increase in blood flow to the brain. Diminished blood flow to the brain is one reason people develop impaired memory and thinking as they get older. Could estrogen prevent or slow this process? It's a distinct possibility.

In other areas of estrogen research, it was found that daily estrogen use can significantly lower blood pressure in post-menopausal women. Healthy post-menopausal women without high blood pressure were given a sequential estrogen/progesterone treatment for one year. At the end of the year, blood pressure was significantly lower in women using estrogen compared to those who did not. The decrease in blood pressure was equal to the benefits of some popular blood pressure medications such as verapamil (Verelan, Calan, Isoptin).

Testosterone Replacement for Men

"I just found out through my V.A. doctor that my testosterone levels should be in the 220s and mine is in the 70s (I'm 49 yrs old). I have osteoarthritis, fibromyalgia, numbness in upper legs, and lately my left nipple has been very painful. I had a mammogram that came back okay, thank God. So now the doctor thinks that this is why I have Chronic Fatigue Syndrome. Will my energy come back to me after I start using the testosterone patches? I can hardly get out of bed for very long at all, and I am hoping this will help me have a better life.

Dennis

Testosterone, the primary hormone produced by the testicle, promotes most of the masculine characteristics of the body. These include development of the penis in fetuses and later, increased muscle strength and muscle mass, facial and body hair, and male sexual function. When testosterone levels are low, it can lead to loss of energy, depression, thinning of the bone (osteoporosis), loss of sexual interest and function and muscle wasting.

There are many medical conditions in men that result in hypogonadism or low testosterone levels (usually in the low 200s or slightly less), so the first challenge is having the condition properly diagnosed. Testosterone levels in men typically decline with aging and by the age of 60 about 20% of men have low testosterone levels. This type of hypogonadism, which develops due to aging, is sometimes

called 'andropause'; this is known to be the male version of menopause. However, aging isn't the only culprit. Trauma to the testicles
such as sports injuries or mumps, tumors of the pituitary gland or
even prolonged and severe illnesses can all cause low testosterone
levels. Another common cause of low testosterone is a failure of the
pituitary gland to make enough of the hormones that cause the testicles to manufacture testosterone. In almost all of these cases the
pituitary gland appears otherwise normal.

Testosterone Replacement Options

Once a low testosterone level is detected and if there is no revers-
ible cause of this problem, then testosterone replacement is generally
advised. The use of an injection to administer testosterone was the
first method used to boost testosterone levels and was fairly common
until the last decade or so. However, the injections, which are given
every two or three weeks, cause a rapid increase of testosterone to
unnaturally high levels followed by steady decline often to low levels again before the next shot. Since testosterone levels are naturally
constant from day to day, this really isn't the best way to mimic naturally occurring testosterone levels.

Based on the shortcomings of injections, testosterone-containing
patches and gels have been developed that can be applied to the skin.
This way the hormone is continuously absorbed through the skin
into the bloodstream. Among the first preparations designed for skin
application was Testoderm, which employs a testosterone-containing patch applied directly to the testicle. Due to inconvenience and
discomfort this product has not been very popular. Another patch

is Androderm, which can be placed on any area of skin on the body that is free of hair. The adhesive on the patch occasionally causes a skin rash, and the patch itself is cumbersome. Up to one third of individuals using a testosterone patch experience some discomfort.

An easy way to avoid the inconvenience and irritation of a patch is to use a testosterone gel like Androgel or Testim. The gel is rubbed directly into the skin every day, making it the easiest and least irritating way to get testosterone into the body through the skin. Studies have shown high levels of patient satisfaction with the gel product. In a study conducted at Duke University, researchers found that men with testosterone levels less than 300 ng/dl treated with Androgel (testosterone gel) had significant improvement in sexual function, muscle strength and lean body mass. Overall satisfaction was better with Androgel than with the testosterone patch.

There are pros and cons to all three treatment methods, but I find most patients tend to prefer the gel. The gel should rub in and mostly disappear, although at higher doses a 'greasy" residue may be left. Everyone is different so you may prefer one type of application to the other but you can get the same levels of testosterone with either method. Be sure to talk to your doctor about your preferences.

Benefits of Testosterone Replacement

Most people think about testosterone replacement as a way to improve symptoms like moodiness, fatigue, weakness, low motivation and loss of sexual interest and function. However, testosterone replacement may help in other important areas of a man's health.

Testosterone is a powerful anti-inflammatory. In the lab it has been shown to suppress the action of chemicals that promote inflammation while upping the effects of powerful anti-inflammatory molecules. This has a number of applications in the prevention and treatment of disease. First, there are several reports of using testosterone therapy to treat inflammatory conditions like rheumatoid arthritis and lupus. Also, since inflammation is a key player in the development and progression of heart disease, testosterone may be important for preventing blood vessel damage and deadly heart attacks.

A number of research studies have shown that men with low testosterone levels are at increased risk of developing coronary artery disease. In a review of 30 different studies, 18 found low testosterone levels in men diagnosed with heart disease. This may be because low testosterone levels are linked to many of the things that put men at a much higher risk of developing heart disease, such as high blood pressure, high "bad" cholesterol levels and low "good" cholesterol levels.

Potential Risks

There are several concerns men often have about taking testosterone supplements. One of the biggest is cancer.

"I'm 43, and I have all symptoms of low testosterone. I'm irritable. When I come home from work I'm spent. I have started to gain weight fast even though I work out and watch what I eat. Depression and forgetfulness has started to creep in. Every joint in my body hurts even though I have been through every

blood test out there (PSA, rheumatoid arthritis, viruses, even thyroid) and the only thing found was low testosterone. My sex life is so-so. I have sex but it's not as fulfilling and erections are not as hard as they should be and I'm losing desire for my wife. My test results are 230 and 1.04, but my doctor is wary of giving me testosterone because in his words: 'It's a very powerful drug, and I'm just not sure about giving it to you.' So he is sending me to an endocrinologist which will take almost 60 days to get an appointment. My question is: My dad and grandfather both had prostate cancer (both survived). I get the PSA regularly and mine is fine, but should I worry about getting testosterone replacement if they actually decide give it to me?"

Terry

Although testosterone probably does not cause cancer to develop within the prostate, it will promote the growth of prostate cancers that otherwise may have been inactive. For this reason, once you start testosterone replacement therapy your PSA levels should be monitored and your prostate should be examined regularly. Excessive amounts of testosterone may also cause breast enlargement (gynecomastia) due to the body's conversion of excess testosterone to estrogen. Aggressive behavior may be promoted as well. When an optimal dose is used, though, testosterone replacement can make a substantial contribution to the well being of men with low testosterone levels.

Human Growth Hormone in Adults

Growth hormone is a protein-based hormone made by the pituitary gland that is probably best known for its role in promoting normal growth in children. Growth hormone controls the liver's production of IGF (insulin like growth factor), formerly known as somatomedin, which stimulates the growth of cartilage. In turn, this results in increasing the size of our bones. Once the bone has finished growing and the growth plates have "closed" or "fused," though, the use of growth hormone no longer increases bone length or height. However, this doesn't mean that growth hormone stops playing an important role in the body.

There are many tissues in the body that have "receptors" for HGH so it has become clear that growth hormone continues to have multiple functions once we have fully grown to our adult size. It plays a role in maintenance of bone, muscles, the brain, immune cells and other tissues. I believe that nature intended growth hormones to maintain, sustain and repair the body that it helped create during the development years. Without them, the aging process causes cell death, starvation and disrepair with no way of regenerating new cells. Therefore they help ward off decline and death.

Growth hormone naturally circulates in our blood in abundant amounts during the first twenty years of our lives but levels slowly decline as we get older. In fact, researchers have calculated that growth hormone levels decline by 14% per decade in adults.

The decline in growth hormone levels associated with aging is mirrored by a decline in a host of other critical substances that help maintain our health, such as DHEA (from the adrenal gland). One possible reason for the drop in these beneficial substances is the plain and simple purpose of promoting our aging and eventual death. The survival of our species requires the removal of the old genetic material (us) so it can be replaced by the new (and possibly improved) genetic material of our offspring. Aging and death are required by the laws of evolution, and therefore our bodies are programmed to self-destruct. The decline in growth hormone may be one way to serve this purpose.

Confirming this theory is a recent study conducted in the Netherlands and UK that was published in the *Journal of Endocrinology and Metabolism*. The researchers compared the body mass index (BMI), waist circumference, triglycerides and HDL (good cholesterol), between normal adults and those with low growth hormone levels due to low pituitary function (hypopituitarism). The results showed that all of the measures were significantly worse in adults younger than 57 years with growth hormone deficiency compared to normal adults of a similar age. The authors noted that the effect of growth hormone deficiency on the bodies of these adults was equivalent to about 40 years of aging! The theory that growth hormone helps preserve our tissues during youth and that aging results from its absence appears to be confirmed by these results.

Diagnosing Growth Hormone Deficiency

If I suspect one of my patients of having growth hormone deficiency based on their history and physical exam, I check their levels of morning growth hormone and IGF. If their growth hormone is in the low-normal range (below 2) the next step is a stimulation test to see whether their pituitary gland can be forced to release its store of the hormone. There are several tests that stimulate the pituitary release of growth hormone, but the simplest is to administer L-dopa (a prescription drug formerly used to treat Parkinson's disease) by mouth and measure growth hormone levels in the blood over the next 2 hours. If the level remains below 5, a growth hormone deficiency can be diagnosed. Many insurance companies will not accept the L-Dopa test alone, as proof of growth hormone deficiency. Without additional confirmation the insurance company will not pay for growth hormone treatment which can be as much as $15,000 per year.

Other acceptable growth hormone stimulation tests are conducted by giving intravenous arginine or an injection of glucagon, both of which have a brief but potent growth hormone elevating effect. If the growth hormone level does not increase above 3 then growth hormone deficiency is confirmed.

Benefits of Growth Hormone Supplementation

Despite its link to reducing aging and a host of other harmful bodily changes, the use of growth hormone supplements in adults remains controversial (due to the potential for abuse and high cost). Recent editorials in the prestigious *New England Journal of Medicine* have taken a negative view of growth hormone supplementation for adults. Dr. Mary Lee Vance commented that the "general use (of growth hormone therapy in adults) now or in the immediate future is not justified."

However, I disagree. I have seen impressive improvements in mood and energy in my adult patients treated with low doses of growth hormone. It is hard to measure these effects, but statements such as: *"Growth hormone changed the quality of my life. The strength and energy I used to have is back in full"* have been used by patients to describe their results.

Like any treatment, there is the potential for side effects. Minor joint pains, carpal tunnel like symptoms, headache, and traces of swelling at the ankle have been described. Unfortunately, experts such as those quoted in the *New England Journal of Medicine* use ominous tones when referring to growth hormone side effects or to the possibility of it causing cancer or cardiovascular disease. These warnings have no data from clinical trials to back them up. In my practice, I generally follow a year or two of treatment with growth hormone followed by 6 months off, just in case there is any possibility of accumulating negative effects of long-term growth hormone therapy.

The medical community is still waiting for the official verdict on growth hormone therapy in adults, but based on reputable studies and my own observations I will continue to offer this treatment to my patients who show the signs, symptoms and blood test evidence of low growth hormone. As with any medical treatment, it is important for each individual to consult with his or her own doctor before embarking on any course of therapy.

Adrenal Fatigue: Fact or Fiction?

The adrenal glands sit on top of the kidneys and make several hormones critical to life. The central part of the adrenal glands make the catecholamine hormones we refer to as adrenalin. These hormones are made in response to stress and cause a rapid heart rate, sweating, increased mental alertness, thus preparing the body for "fight or flight." The outer portion of the adrenal gland makes the hormone cortisol, also known as cortisone. Cortisol maintains, among other things, blood pressure and fluid and salt balance. Without sufficient cortisol production by the adrenals, life cannot be sustained.

"Adrenal fatigue" is a recently proposed diagnosis used to explain a variety of general symptoms such as fatigue, moodiness, muscle aches and diminished mental function. Supposedly, adrenal fatigue results from mild impairment of cortisol production. There are no scientific studies supporting the notion that this form of adrenal fatigue exists. Worse than being a bogus diagnosis is that practitioners are prescribing steroids like prednisone as treatment for "adrenal fatigue".

I need to point out, that adrenal hormones are so crucial to maintaining basic life functions that if the adrenals actually did fatigue, it wouldn't cause minor complaints like tiredness or muscle aches; it would put you in the ICU or outright kill you. Additionally, the recommended treatment breaks every rule in the medical books, since steroid use is universally held to an absolute minimum to avoid devastating complications like defective immune function, bleeding stomach ulcer, thinning of the skin, abdominal obesity, wasting of the muscles and mood disorders like depression.

I hold a very dim view of the practitioners who propose to diagnose and treat adrenal fatigue. My advice to them is to drop the charade and get on with helping people in legitimate ways.

Conclusion

Your metabolism and your hormones are two of the biggest factors affecting your health and wellbeing. As a result, when they are screwed up or out of balance, the world seems like it is not well. Unfortunately, many people find that getting these problems under control is a struggle—both inside themselves and against the mainstream medical establishment.

Therefore it is important for you to know that you are not alone. There are other people out there who are dealing with the same issues you are and are searching for the same solutions.

I hope you have found this eBook to be helpful and that it has answered many of the questions you may have had about the wide range of problems related to metabolism, nutritional health and weight control, as well as conditions such as diabetes and thyroid disorders. If you are still searching for answers or would like more information on any of the topics covered in this book, I encourage you to visit Metabolism.com and interact with the amazing collection of members and experts who gather there.

"I recently went to hear your broadcast and wanted you to know how grateful we are to know that you exist and are willing to stand up for what you have found to be quality care for your patients. Truly, the lack of concern and rigid indifference that many specialists have for the suffering of those who trust them is shameful. However we are all human, and we all resist change. Please remain vocal. You are in a unique position to have a voice. I can imagine that it takes courage and, strong self-esteem to be a "lone wolf." Just know that we truly appreciate your efforts."

Lil

"Thank you so much for providing sound alternatives and such clear guidance on the whys of it all. I, and I'm sure many more, thank you!"

Lynette

The Birth Of Metabolism.com

I first conceived the idea for Metabolism.com around 1994. At the time I was Chief of the Division of Endocrinology for New York Medical College based at Lincoln Hospital and Medical Center. Lincoln is a city run hospital located in the South Bronx, and at that time it was an epicenter of the AIDS epidemic and diseases like tuberculosis. Eight years prior to my arrival, it was also the place where the movie Fort Apache was filmed, depicting life at the 41st Police Precinct in the middle of an urban wasteland. Despite the limitations of that situation, professionally it was a good time for me.

With one or two other physician attendings and our endocrinologists in training (Fellows) we ran the service responsible for all the endocrine health problems of this immense and underserved community. We saw a lot, did a lot and felt good about what we were doing. I also built a respectable laboratory and collaborated with other doctors and scientists, a privilege few other physicians can claim to have had. Because I didn't have a private practice I could focus on academics and look into areas I otherwise might not have had time for.

One thing that appealed to me was the growing Internet community and computer-based technologies. Wouldn't it be great to reach a really large audience with health care information? I had no idea I was on the threshold of a cultural revolution but I was one of many who felt the growing excitement. My other responsibilities limited just how much I could do with this interest, however.

Two years later I reserved the domain name, Metabolism.com and began a 15 year journey. At first I did all my own programming and was the sole contributor. It was fun! Google didn't exist and there was no organized way for people to find me, but the name "Metabolism. com" itself brought some visitors. My dream was to bring together all varieties of experts within the field of metabolism and nutrition in one place so that a visitor could access a nutritionist, endocrinologist, herbalist, aromatherapy expert etc. I was to be the moderator.

The biggest obstacle other than having no cash and my own lack of business experience was that no one trusted me! There was so much publicity surrounding the new Internet millionaires with their get-rich-quick schemes that the professionals I wanted to bring to the website thought I was going to exploit them. At first I was confused by the cold reception because I thought I was giving them a highly visible place to practice their art and science.

I did attract a few professionals including the nutritionist Dr. Robert Pastore, who at the time was just starting up his practice as a nutritionist. I paid him very little but he was so enthusiastic and full of energy he just carried on and built a nice following. Eventually his own practice in New York City got too big and he left Metabolism.com. Others followed but generally the demands on their professional and personal time led to rapid turnover of my collaborators. Reluctantly I gave up on the idea of being a "clearing house" for experts in metabolism and health.

Others with similar concepts have succeeded to some degree but I am not impressed with many of these websites because they seem stiflingly "corporate" or exist only to sell a product. Some sites are based on a single bogus principle, geared to making someone with few qualifications into a guru for a non-existent disease.

My Path Into Endocrinology

I didn't know I wanted to be an endocrinologist until relatively late in my medical training. Endocrinology as a specialty was relatively new and until I had learned a fair bit about medicine, I didn't even know what endocrinology was. The first role model for my future career was Harold Rifkin, M.D. a noted diabetes expert. He was my teacher (attending) when I was an intern at Montefiore Hospital in the Bronx, N.Y., (a part of Albert Einstein School of Medicine).

A young man with type 1 diabetes was admitted to our medical service because he was having episodes of fainting, low blood pressure and extreme fatigue. He even fainted in the shower while he was a patient in the hospital (come to think of it, if that was now he probably would have sued me and Dr. Rifkin for that). He also had unexpectedly high potassium levels. Everyone thought his episodes were due to low blood pressure attacks from dehydration or low blood sugar due to diabetes but I didn't agree. I was suspicious he had Addison's Disease (adrenal insufficiency) since that made sense with all the findings, and I was right. Dr. Rifkin was impressed with me and invited me to his Park Avenue apartment for dinner. My eyes were finally shining after being a lowly trainee for so many years!

I still wasn't prepared to be an endocrinologist, however. Then my dad developed prostate cancer. By the time it was diagnosed it had already spread to his bones and was incurable. There was not much the doctors could do for him. It was known that prostate cancer grows faster in the presence of the male hormone, testosterone. Removing testosterone causes prostate cancer to halt in its tracks, at least for a few years. Back then, the only way to achieve this was to perform an orchiectomy or removal of the testicles, a procedure my father underwent. Immediately the pain in his bone ceased and he returned to normal for the next 5 years, until the tumor started growing again. My fascination with hormones was solidified by this experience.

As my interest in endocrinology grew as an intern and resident at Montefiore, I had the fortune to train with Dr. Martin Surks. Dr. Surks is one of the pioneers of thyroid science, has written innumerable publications on the subject and is one of the founders of the American Thyroid Association (ATA). He offered me a fellowship at Montefiore but I had my sights set on Mt. Sinai in Manhattan, reputed to be the best endocrine training center in the East. That's where I met Dr. Dorothy Krieger.

Dr. Krieger, Chief of Endocrinology at Mt. Sinai, was driven to succeed more than anyone I had ever met. It seemed to me that every second of her life was devoted to science, writing grants and climbing the academic ladder. She didn't bother with good morning, how are you etc. In fact, she wasn't very nice at all. But what an intellect!!

Just as I was starting my fellowship with her, a young brash English endocrinologist, Terry Davies, M.D., joined Dr. Krieger's department. Terry has spent his entire career trying to understand how the immune system affects the thyroid gland. Terry was in many ways the opposite of Dr. Krieger because he was approachable and kind.

But the person who impressed me most was Kenneth Davis, M.D. He had just been made head of the psychiatry department at the Bronx VA hospital, which was affiliated with Mt. Sinai. Already a renown neuropharmacologist, he was leading the search for a connection between brain chemicals (neurotransmitters), hormones and behavior. This was also one of the main interests of Dr. Krieger. I was present at the first meeting of Ken Davis and Krieger and was responsible for settling him into her office to wait for her. He was curious about what sort of person she was, and eager to learn any little tid bits I could offer about working with her. I guess I was too honest, as is my fault. I don't know for sure but I don't think that initial meeting went too well.

Another big mistake I made was to tell Dr. Krieger I wanted to work for Ken Davis rather than her. I wanted to learn more about the brain, hormones and behavior, and Dr. Davis was willing to let me work on some of my own ideas. Dr. Krieger would have none of that sort of thing. Terry Davies subsequently told me that after that I was on her black list.

I stayed on with Dr. Krieger until the end of my fellowship, writing a chapter in a book, *The Neurobiology of Mood Disorders*, edited by the leaders of neuropharmacology at the NIH. It was a compromise but not nearly as dynamic an experience working with Dr. Ken Davis would have been. Dr. Krieger died tragically a few years later at the age of 58 and Ken Davis is now the President and CEO of Mt. Sinai Medical Center in New York City.

Recent Contributors On Metabolism.com

Over the years I have worked with a great number of highly qualified professionals on the website. Here is a rundown on the most recent active participants.

Beth Ellen DiLuglio, M.S., R.D., C.C.N., LD/N.
Beth Ellen DiLuglio is a Certified Clinical Nutritionist and Registered Dietitian with certification in nutrition support. She earned a Bachelor's in Biology/Psychology from Wheaton College in Norton, Massachusetts before earning a Master of Science degree in Human Nutrition from Columbia University in New York City. More recently, Beth Ellen has developed NutritionMission.org, a web-based resource center that highlights the role of nutrition in disease prevention and risk reduction. She has also provided her services to several not-for-profit agencies and continues to volunteer her services in the quest for disease reduction and health promotion nationwide.

Maya Sarkisyan is a Certified Hypnotist, Master NLP Practitioner, and Master of Acupuncture specializing in Five Element tradition. She has an extensive experience in the various areas of body/mind/spirit healing modalities.

APPENDIX 1

Personal Nutrition Profile

The Personalized Nutrition Profile (PNP for short) is a personalized weight loss program that was designed by the staff at Metabolism.com and offered as a paid service from 2000 until 2007. Because it was personalized, no two PNPs were exactly alike. However, here is an example of a plan that was tailor made for a member named Evelyn who was interested in losing 15-20 pounds and getting proper nutrition. After completing a health assessment questionnaire, a certified nutritionist at Metabolism.com sent Evelyn this detailed PNP. While the recommendations reflect the personal opinions of the nutritionist, they are in alignment with the overall principles of Metabolism.com.

Health Assessment

A balanced nutrition and exercise program can help you reach your goals. Weight control is extremely important in helping to avoid many health conditions down the road, such as the risk of developing cardio-vascular disease, high blood pressure, diabetes and some cancers. You can lose weight and boost your metabolism by performing aerobic and strength training exercises and eating the correct amount of calories in the proper ratios of carbohydrates, proteins and fats. Maintaining a desirable weight is important for long-term good health.

Unfortunately, metabolism slows down with age, resulting in weight gain. It takes a combination of both aerobic and weight bearing ex-ercises to increase metabolism and lose weight. However, in order to see results you need to monitor your caloric intake. Consuming too many calories is detrimental to weight loss. Consuming too few calories will slow the metabolism. The correct food intake, combined with a higher metabolic rate brought about by exercise, can result in the breakdown of fat stores, thus maintaining a lower body weight.

I understand your frustration about trying to lose weight unsuc-cessfully. You mentioned that when you worked out at the gym, you gained or maintained weight. When working out, weight becomes distributed differently in the body. As you build muscle, your weight on the scale will remain the same or even increase, as muscle weighs more than fat. However, you'll notice that clothes start to fit more loosely and you feel better. Stick with your program and make sure to include aerobic as well as strength-training activities. I will cover this later in your Profile under Exercise.

While there is no treatment that directly reverses the impaired glucose tolerance you mentioned, there are, in fact, natural ways to combat it—through diet and exercise. Your Personal Nutrition Profile is designed to include a balanced diet program and exercise guidelines to help boost your metabolic rate so you can reach your weight loss goals. Nutritional information and health tips are also provided to aid you in your quest for overall health and wellness.

BMI/Calorie Analysis

Using your height of 5'3" and your current weight of 133 lbs, I calculated your BMI (Body Mass Index). BMI is a measurement of a person's weight in relation to their height. The normal range is between 19 and 24.9. Your BMI is 23.4, which indicates you are at the higher end of the healthy range. Losing about 20 pounds would bring you to the lower end of the normal range (20), which will be a healthier level for you.

Based on this information, your target caloric intake should be about 1,250 calories per day. This should result in gradual and healthy weight loss. I don't recommend eating less than this amount as you may feel deprived and lack energy, which may result in you giving up on your new lifestyle program. Eating too few calories can also slow the metabolism.

Meal Planning

Now that you have a caloric total to aim for, I have analyzed the proper macronutrient percentages for you to follow. I recommend that approximately 55% of your total calories come from carbohydrates, 20% from proteins, and 25% from healthy, unsaturated fats. This is a good place to start, as eating foods in these percentages will keep your metabolism boosted to aid in fat loss.

A 1,250 calorie/day meal plan consists of:

Complex carbohydrates	5 servings
Protein	2 servings
Vegetables	3-4 servings
Fruits	2 servings
Dairy	1-2 servings
Fats	2 servings

The following Sample Menu offers suggestions for breakfast, lunch, and dinner. If your schedule permits, it's a good idea to break up these meals into four or five smaller meals throughout the day to keep your blood sugar levels steady, avoid hunger pangs, and keep your metabolism running high. It's also important to never skip a meal. Another important note—you should try to stick mainly to whole foods. Try keeping foods in their original state. Minimal processing preserves the nutrients and avoids excess calories and additives. When this is followed, weight loss usually occurs automatically.

You'll notice that for the most part, I've combined carbohydrates with proteins. This is imperative for blood sugar control. Combining carbohydrates with proteins will result in a slower rise in blood sugar, creating satiety. I believe that combining your foods in this manner will help you with your sensitivity to carbohydrates.

Below the Sample Menu I've included food lists to help you avoid having to count calories. Just select the foods you like and insert them into the Sample Menu. Remember to follow the suggested serving sizes.

Sample Menu

BREAKFAST	LUNCH
½ bagel *(carb)*	½ med. apple *(fruit)*
3 egg whites *(protein)*	1 cup spinach *(vegetable)*
½ cup orange juice *(fruit)*	2 tsp. low or non-fat
¼ cup yogurt *(dairy)*	mayonnaise *(fats)*
	2 oz. sliced turkey *(protein)*
	2 slices whole wheat bread *(carb)*

DINNER	DESSERT
2 oz. chicken *(protein)*	1½" square angel food
1 tsp. salad dressing on endive	cake *(carb)*
lettuce *(vegetable + fat)*	
1 cup broccoli *(vegetable)*	
1/3 cup brown rice *(carb)*	

Complex Carbohydrates

Foods such as breads, cereals and starchy vegetables are considered complex carbohydrates. Remember to choose high fiber foods. Foods high in fiber are digested more slowly, causing a slower rise in blood sugar. Since you are carbohydrate sensitive, it's important to keep in mind to eat less refined starches and sugars and more whole grain foods.

NOTE: The most important thing about carbohydrates is how much you eat. If you eat more carbohydrates than usual, you may not have enough insulin available to transport the excess sugar into your cells, causing an increase in your blood sugar level. One way you can help control your blood sugar is by eating the same amount of carbohydrates at similar times throughout the day.

Rice—1/3 cup cooked

Oats—1/3 cup

Quinoa—½ cup

Bread sticks—3

Graham crackers—(2) 2 ½" squares

Matzo—½

Melba toast (small)—5

Multi-grain bread—1 slice

Oyster crackers—½ cup

Pretzels (unsalted)—8 rings or 3 twists

Rye crisps—3

Saltines (unsalted)—5

Baked potato—½ large

Corn (kernels)—½ cup

Garbanzo / chick peas—½ cup

Legumes (lentils, peas)—½ cup

Potato (mashed)—½ cup

Sweet potato—½ large

Beans (kidney, lima, pinto)—½ cup

Pumpkin—½ cup

Proteins

This category includes fish, poultry, and other lean proteins. You will notice that some of these foods also appear in other categories. When that happens, count the foods listed in more than one category as a serving from each.

Beans, lentils—½ cup

Egg whites—3

Fish (filet)—2 oz

Lobster—1 small tail

Tofu—3 oz

Tuna (in water)—½ cup

Salmon (grilled/canned)—2 oz

Scallops—2 oz.

Oysters, clams, shrimp—5 medium

Skinless poultry (chicken or turkey)—2 oz

Vegetables

Vegetables are an excellent source of vitamins, minerals, and fiber. They are high in nutritional value and low in calories. These servings should be eaten as follows: ½ cup cooked or 1 cup raw.

Artichoke	Asparagus	Beans, green
Beets	Broccoli	Brussels sprouts
Cabbage	Carrots	Cauliflower
Celery	Cucumber	Eggplant
Green onion	Kale	Leeks
Lettuce	Mushrooms	Onions
Parsley	Peppers	Pumpkin
Radishes	Sauerkraut	Snow peas
Spinach	Squash	Tomatoes
Tomato paste	Tomato juice	Turnips
Vegetable juice	Watercress	Zucchini

Fruits

Fruits are also an excellent source of vitamins, minerals, and fiber. They are especially healthy and satisfying for a dessert because they are naturally sweet and contain no fat, and will satisfy your desire for sugary foods.

Apple—½ med.	Apple cider or juice—½ cup
Applesauce (no sugar)—½ cup	Apricots—4 medium-sized, fresh
Blueberries—¾ cup	Cantaloupe—1/3
Cherries—12 large	Cranberry juice—½ cup
Dates—2-1/2 fresh	Figs—2 fresh or 1-1/2 dried
Fruit preserves—2 tsp	Grapes—15
Grape juice—1/3 cup	Grapefruit—½
Grapefruit juice—½ cup	Honeydew melon—¼ medium
Kiwi fruit—1 large	Lemon—1 large
Mango—½ small	Nectarine—1 medium
Orange—1 medium	Orange juice—½ cup
Papaya—½ medium	Peach—1 medium
Pineapple juice—½ cup	Prunes—3 medium
Prune juice—1/3 cup	Raisins—2 Tbsp
Raspberries—¾ cup	Strawberries—¾ cup

Dairy

Dairy products are rich in vitamins, minerals, and protein. However, whole dairy products are high in fat, so be sure to choose non-fat varieties.

Non-fat buttermilk—½ to ¾ cup

Non-fat cheese—3 oz

Non-fat yogurt—½ to ¾ cup

Skim milk—¾ cup

Non-fat cottage cheese—½ cup

Fats

Use these foods only as recommended.

Avocado—1/8

Bacon—1 lean slice

Olive oil—1 tsp

Peanuts—10

Light cream cheese—1 Tbsp

Peanut butter—1 tsp

Butter (no salt or low salt)—1 tsp

Salad dressing—1 tsp (non-fat—1 Tbsp)

Mayonnaise (low fat)—1 tsp (non-fat—1 Tbsp)

Snack Foods

These snack foods can be consumed in unlimited quantities.

Clear broth (low or no salt)	Bouillon
Mustard	Gelatin (sugar-free)
Tea (herbal, caffeine-free)	Vegetable juice
Vinegar	

Spices

Spices can greatly enhance the flavor of many dishes without adding extra fat or calories. Try using basil, chives, curry, ginger, nutmeg, marjoram, oregano, parsley, sage and thyme to spice up your meals. Best of all, using spices and herbs adds flavor without adding sodium or fat.

Beverages

Drinking water is important for overall good health. Water is critical in regulating all body organs and temperature as well as dissolving solids and moving nutrients throughout the body. Research has shown that proper hydration may minimize chronic pains such as rheumatoid arthritis, lower back pain, migraines and colitis, as well as helping lower cholesterol and blood pressure.

I suggest that you consume a <u>minimum</u> of 8 to 10 eight-ounce glasses of water per day. When you exercise, you'll want to consume more than the recommended amount. If in doubt of how much water you consumed, drink some more! Quality, filtered water is the best

METABOLISM

choice although you can incorporate caffeine-free herbal teas and seltzer. Caffeinated beverages, as well as alcohol, should be avoided as they can cause the body to lose water. Also, avoid diet soft drinks as they can signal a craving for carbohydrates.

Nutritional Supplements

Although you may try to eat a healthy diet, there are some nutrients that are either lacking from the diet or are in short supply. For example, vitamin E is found in vegetable oils, nuts and seeds, wheat germ, and dark leafy greens. However, you'd need to eat 25 pounds of almonds or consume nearly nine cups of canola oil to get 400 IUs, the "heart healthy" recommended intake! Judging by the supplement program you currently follow, I can see that you certainly understand why supplementation is important.

I suggest that you continue taking the nutritional supplements you mentioned on the questionnaire (multi-vitamin and calcium/magnesium). Make sure that the calcium supplement you take contains vitamin D and/or boron to aid absorption. Take 1,200 milligrams in divided doses between meals daily. Also, taking it at night may help you sleep.

Some other nutrients that you may find helpful are:

- *Digestive Enzymes/HCl (Hydrochloric acid)*—These will help break down food and release vitamins, minerals and amino acids. If your body is not digesting food properly, you are missing out on vital nutrient absorption. Take digestive enzymes and

HCl before or after meals (may be taken several times a day, as needed).

- *GTF chromium*—Studies show that GTF (glucose tolerance factor), which contains chromium, helps make insulin work better by naturally lowering blood sugar levels. GTF is an essential micronutrient found naturally in many foods, but many people are deficient. It may be helpful for you to take 200 mcg daily.

- *Gymnema sylvestre and fenugreek*—Some studies show that these herbs can help reduce sugar cravings and lower blood sugar levels. Begin with at least 400 mg each daily; you can increase the amount to 2 grams daily, if desired.

- *Valerian root*—This herb can help relax the central nervous system, aiding in sleep. Take approximately 500 mg an hour before bedtime.

Keeping a Journal

Writing down your goals in a journal can be very helpful in reaching them. When goals are written out, they tend to be adhered to more closely. Seeing your goals written out will keep you focused as you review your journal daily.

It's also a good idea to create a food journal to help you keep track of the foods you eat, when you eat them, and in what quantities. I suggest you write out a basic menu of what you intend to eat throughout the next month. Using the above guidelines, take a calendar and write out your food plan. Following your food plan will help keep you on track towards reaching your weight-loss goal. It also makes grocery shopping easier when you know basically what you are going to eat over the next month. Buying the healthy foods on your menu will keep the junk food out of your home. If the junk food's not there, you won't eat it!

To help you out a food journal is included in *Appendix 3*. Feel free to make copies and use it to help keep track of your dietary intake. When everything is written out, it makes tracking your progress easier. You can see where you need to make adjustments in diet or exercise to reach your goals.

Exercise

As you know, exercise is a very important part of weight loss and a healthy lifestyle. For the best results with weight loss and jump-starting the metabolism, you need to perform aerobic and strength-training activities. **Always check with your doctor before beginning any exercise program.**

Walking is a very effective form of cardiovascular activity. Although walking is low in intensity, it still burns fat over a longer period of time. Walking not only burns calories, it improves your circulation, helps strengthen your bones, builds and maintains muscle mass, and helps relieve stress. Another bonus: during exercise your metabolic rate will increase and remain elevated for several hours afterward.

Exercising can be fun! When the weather outside is nice, go for a walk. During inclement weather, perhaps your local gym or YWCA has treadmills available for use at a nominal cost. Just begin slowly and work your way up. Begin with 10 minutes per day at a moderate pace. Gradually increase the number of minutes per day until you reach 30 minutes at least five times a week. (Walking at 2 mph for 30 minutes will burn approximately 127 calories.) When you reach this level, gradually pick up the pace and increase the intensity to burn more calories. **If any unusual chest pain or shortness of breath occurs, stop exercising and consult your physician immediately.** Make sure to warm up and cool down before and after exercise to prevent injury. And don't forget to drink <u>lots</u> of water!

Strength training is helpful for supporting muscle growth and maintenance. The more muscle mass you have, the more calories you will burn. As a start, you may want to purchase your own set of dumbbells and begin lifting weights at home. If you want to join a gym, most have a circuit-training setup where you can move from machine to machine, each one working a different muscle group. If possible, you may want to look into getting a personal trainer who can give you proper instruction and help you develop a weight-lifting program that works best for you.

Exercise should also be noted somewhere in your journal. Note when you exercise, the length of time, intensity, and how often you exercise.

Tips

Here are some tips I have found helpful for weight maintenance. I hope you find them helpful, too! Remembering the portion sizes comes in handy when you dine out.

When eating in a restaurant, try to stick to healthy choices. Forego the bread and butter, the sour cream and butter on a baked potato, cream soups, cream sauces, etc. For example, baked or broiled chicken or fish is the best option for an entrée with steamed vegetables and wild rice on the side. Portion sizes can be kept under control by following these simple guidelines:

- Three ounces of cooked meat, poultry, or fish is about the size of a deck of cards or the palm of a small woman's hand.
- One cup of cooked rice or vegetables is about the size of a small fist.
- One ounce of cheese is about the size of four stacked dice.
- One teaspoon of mayonnaise, peanut butter or salad dressing is about the size of the tip of your thumb, from the tip to the knuckle.
- One ounce of nuts or raisins is the amount you can hold in your cupped hand, if you have a small hand.

The calories can really stack up with larger portions than these. An extra 250 calories per day adds up to two addition pounds each month. That's 24 pounds in a year! So make sure to follow these guidelines to reach your weight loss goals.

Final Notes

All of this information can be overwhelming at first. So you may find it helpful to review everything several times to understand all the aspects of your new healthy lifestyle program. Once you get used to your new program, it will become second nature to you.

Please make an extra copy of your Personal Nutrition Profile and post it somewhere where you can see it regularly! There is too much information here to remember it all. Reviewing your program regularly will help you continue with your new healthy routine.

APPENDIX 2

Ultimate Weight Gain Program

Many Metabolism.com members want to gain weight in a healthy manner. As a result, the certified nutritionists at Metabolism.com developed a personalized weight gain program and offered it as a paid service. Because it was personalized, no two programs were exactly alike. However, here is an example of a plan that was tailor made for a member named Brandy. After completing a health assessment questionnaire, a certified nutritionist at Metabolism.com developed this detailed program for Brandy. While the recommendations reflect the personal opinions of the nutritionist, they are in alignment with the overall principles of Metabolism.com.

BMI/Calorie Analysis

Using your height of 5'11" and your current weight of 125 lbs, I calculated your BMI (Body Mass Index). BMI is a measurement of a person's weight in relation to their height. Your BMI is 17.4. The normal range is between 18 and 24.9. However, this measurement tool is not completely accurate when it comes to certain individuals. For example, almost all professional athletes, from long-distance runners to professional body builders, have very high BMIs. This is because muscle weighs more than fat but occupies less space. So body weight will be much higher in a well-sculpted body builder when compared to one of his/her non-training peers.

Our short-term goal is to increase your BMI by adding muscle, and our long-term goal is to strive to increase your weight and level of muscle development. Based on this information, our target caloric total should be about 2,500 calories per day. I chose this caloric total for several reasons. First, I use a standard formula that is used heavily in clinical research for Basal Metabolic Rate called the Harris-Benedict equation. Then I added in your caloric expenditure for your height and weight. Finally, I added additional calories to help you increase muscle mass. (Please refer to my "Notes on Weight Gain" towards the end of this plan.)

Now that we have a caloric total to aim for, we must determine the best macronutrient percentage for your situation. Based on your information, I recommend that 40% of your calories come from carbohydrates and 30% from protein, leaving 30% from fat. Since your diet is intended to assist with muscle growth, we want to make sure you are consuming enough protein to aid in the growth and repair of muscle tissue. Additionally, we need to add plenty of complex carbohydrates. Carbohydrates are essential in a weight-gain and muscle-building program. They provide the energy needed for exercise, plus if eaten in high enough quantities, they provide a "protein sparing" action. This is very important. Many strength trainers can't understand why they aren't gaining muscle when they are consuming plenty of protein. If they are not consuming enough carbohydrates, then the answer lies in a biochemical process called gluconeogenesis (the making of glucose from a non-carbohydrate source). This non-carbohydrate source is inevitably protein, usually muscle protein. Having plenty of carbs in your diet prevents this from occurring and reserves your protein intake for strength training support and muscle growth.

Meal Planning

2,500 calories:

    40% carbohydrates: 1,000 calories or 250 grams

    30% protein: 750 calories or 187 grams

    30% fat: 750 calories or 83 grams

There are two options for your diet pattern:

Option one:

    3 servings "whey" protein and carbohydrate dietary supplement

    7 servings complex carbohydrates from whole grains, starchy vegetables, and beans

    3 servings fruit

4 servings vegetables

3 servings dairy (full fat milk and yogurt)

3 servings protein (each serving should be at least 6 oz)

5 servings fats (1 tsp per serving)

Option two:

2 servings "whey" protein and carbohydrate dietary supplement

7 servings complex carbohydrates from whole grains, starchy vegetables, and beans

3 servings fruit

4 servings vegetables

3 servings dairy (full fat milk and yogurt)

4 servings protein (each serving should be at least 6 oz)

5 servings fats (1 tsp per serving)

The difference between the two is that the whey meal can be used two or three times per day. When it is used three times, you only need three servings of protein. When it is used only two times, your protein intake (meat, poultry, fish, pork) increases to four servings per day.

Here is a sample list of suggestions that you can use to prevent counting calories when trying to plan meals. The key is to choose some of your favorite healthy foods following the suggested servings and insert them into a menu format. You can choose any healthy foods for breakfast, lunch and dinner, and include healthy snacks. The following is only an example to illustrate how quick and easy it can be to obtain all of the above servings over the course of the day, without ever counting calories. These examples can be expanded upon, and the choices vary so much that a cookbook would be needed to depict all the possibilities.

Breakfast Suggestions

An egg white omelet (eight egg whites plus one whole egg) with onions and peppers, two slices of whole grain toast, 1 tsp butter, herbal tea (such as green tea), a glass of regular milk and a piece of fruit.

> NOTE: If you have problems digesting milk or milk products, try using lactose-free milk or take lactase, an enzyme to aid the digestion of lactose.

OR

A shake containing 42 grams of whey protein with one piece of fruit, one cup of regular milk and 1 Tbsp of flax oil

OR

Leftover protein (6 oz of ground meat, turkey, etc.) reheated and served with one cup of rice and the seasonings of your choice

OR

One cup of cooked oatmeal with two scoops of Designer Whey Protein powder

OR

Three scrambled eggs with two turkey sausages and two slices of whole grain toast with butter and 100% fruit spread

Lunch Suggestions

At least 6 oz of fresh turkey on whole grain bread or roll with lettuce and tomato, and a large mixed green and bean salad with olive oil and vinegar dressing (1 tsp).

OR

Six ounces of grilled chicken breast with steamed broccoli and cauliflower (one cup) paired with one cup of lentil soup made with lentils, carrots, olive oil, tomato and your favorite spices.

OR

One can of tuna, made into tuna salad with your favorite additions (whatever vegetables and other ingredients you desire), as well as some carbs, such as brown or white rice, pasta, beans or whole grain crackers

Dinner Suggestions

Baked salmon with lemon and olive oil sauce, steamed vegetable platter (green beans, kale, bok choy), one large sweet potato, 2/3 cup of brown rice, one cup milk, fresh melon for desert.

OR

Six ounces of shrimp, a large green salad (two cups), and one cup of whole grain pasta, with one cup of pinto beans sautéed in 1 tsp of olive oil with your favorite spices, covered in tomato sauce.

OR

Homemade pizza with whole grain prepared pizza crust, 6 oz of cooked ground meat, 6 oz of cheese, tomato sauce and red bell peppers (1/2 cup).

Snack Suggestions

Whey protein shakes (two per day), yogurt, a hand full of mixed dry roasted nuts, a piece of fruit (such as a granny smith apple) with almond nut butter, peanut butter sandwich, one cup of a legume salad, etc.

Here is a conversion chart of serving sizes specifically tailored to your diet. Note that these are not standard serving sizes. They are unique to your plan. Instead of having a frustrating time counting calories, just use your above diet pattern (the list of how many servings per food group) and fill in the serving sizes from those listed below. This will make meal preparation a snap. Remember your goal...you don't want to eat less than what your body needs in order for you to gain weight.

Serving Sizes

Determining the proper serving size isn't always easy. However, the lists below help illustrate serving sizes in a way that will make meeting your dietary requirements much simpler.

Each equals one serving of complex carbohydrates:

　　1 slice whole grain bread

　　1 small whole grain pita

　　½ cup cooked whole grain

　　1 cup ready-to-eat cereal in flake form (Total, corn flakes, etc.)

　　½ whole grain bun, bagel, roll

　　6 small whole grain crackers

　　1 small baked sweet or white potato, 1/2 cup of winter squash

　　½ cup legumes

Each equals one serving of vegetables:

　　1 cup raw vegetables

　　½ cup cooked vegetables

　　3/4 cup vegetable juice

Each equals one serving of fruit:

　　1 piece fruit

　　½ cup dried fruit

　　1 cup juice

　　1 cup berries

　　1 melon wedge

　　20 grapes

METABOLISM.com

Each equals one serving of lean protein:

6 oz cooked chicken, fresh turkey, extra lean sirloin, lean pork or fish

8 egg whites, plus 1 whole egg

6 oz cheese

Each equals one serving of dairy:

8 oz yogurt

8 oz milk

Each equals one serving of fats:

1 tsp butter, canola oil, olive oil, flax oil or salad dressing

1 Tbsp nuts or nut butter

1 Tbsp cream cheese

1 Tbsp seeds (except for flax seeds—3 Tbsp equals 2 servings of fat)

1 whole egg

1 oz low-fat cheese

15 corn chips cooked in oil

NOTE: Six ounces of extra lean sirloin can equal up to five servings of fat. Half of an avocado can equal three servings of fat.

It also important to understand how certain foods crossover into other food groups. For example, you can see that while an egg is a source of protein, but it is also a source of fat. So one whole egg will equal one serving of fat as well as part of your protein component. Additionally, since a serving of oil (a fat) is measured by the teaspoon, we can estimate that one tablespoon equals three servings of fat. Does this mean that you have to count how many egg yolks you eat or measure the size of red meat that you have in order to accurately calculate your fat intake? The answer is absolutely not! I calculated all of your protein, carbohydrate and fat requirements. Just make sure not to eat too little, and be aware of what serving sizes are to prevent that from happening.

Please don't think that you will be counting serving sizes for the rest of your life. This is not the case. Over time as you gain healthy weight, you will begin to realize how much food your body needs and notice that you are actually able to estimate how much you are actually eating without resorting to measuring cups. Like any new information, practice makes perfect. Just practicing measuring out portions will enable you to become more comfortable planning meals and eating out. You will notice that you can "eye" a serving size. Additionally, since we all eat at least three times per day, you will be using this new information on a daily basis, and will notice it will become second nature in no time.

How to Estimate

A quarter pounder and a half is 6 oz. Try to imagine what that would look like in the palm of your hand. If laid flat, it would reach up to your first joint toward the tip of your fingers. To visualize 6 oz, ask a deli worker to weigh 6 oz of turkey breast. Feel the weight and notice the size.

As for grain estimations, a basic serving will look like half a baseball on your plate. You will need to consume much more to meet your calorie total. This can be achieved by consuming more than one serving per meal, as I indicated on the sample menu. A great complex carbohydrate for you would be legumes (beans of any variety). One cup cooked equals two servings. Better yet, one 15-ounce can contains approximately three servings. You can just open a can (Eden is the best) and use the entire contents with your meal (but watch out for the sodium content). For example, turkey chili made with one can of chili beans, 6 oz of turkey and some vegetables would equal three servings of carbohydrates, one serving of protein, and the vegetable component would depend on the amount of vegetables you use. The key is to keep it simple!

Here is a listing of foods that you might want to use when planning your menu:

Protein: Whole egg—try the brand Eggland's Best, which contain higher essential fatty acids, regular organic eggs, or the brand DHA eggs, egg whites (any brand), chicken, turkey, any fish (salmon is an excellent choice), extra lean sirloin, buffalo, lean pork

Dairy protein: Milk, yogurt, cheese (any type)

Whole grains: Amaranth, barley, brown rice, buckwheat, bulgur, corn meal, kamut, millet, oats, rye, spelt, teff, triticale, quinoa, whole wheat, whole grain ready-to-eat dry cereals (any variety)

Refined grains: White rice, pasta (any type), corn chips cooked in healthy oil, breads, rolls, ready-to-eat cereals (low sugar, such as Wheaties or Cheerios)

Legumes: Adzuki, black eyed peas, black turtle beans, garbanzo beans, kidney beans, lentils, lima beans, mung beans, navy beans, peas, pinto beans

Nuts (nut milks, nut butters included): Almonds, cashews, Brazil, filberts, macadamia, pecans, pine, pistachios, walnuts

Seeds (seed butters and pastes included): Flax, pumpkin, sesame, sunflower, tahini

Substitutes: Fortified soymilk may be used as a substitute for regular milk

Non and mildly starchy vegetables: Asparagus, avocado, green/wax beans, beets and beet greens, bok choy, broccoli, Brussels sprouts, cabbage, cauliflower, celery, chard, chicory, collard greens, crookneck squash, cucumber, dandelion, eggplant, endive, escarole, kale, kohlrabi, leek, mushrooms, mustard greens, okra, onion, parsley, parsnips, radishes, romaine lettuce, ruta-baga, scallions, spinach, summer squash, Swiss chard, sprouts, tomato, turnips, watercress, zucchini

Starchy vegetables: Artichoke, carrots, corn, delicata squash, peppers (red, yellow, green), potato (sweet, white, yams) pumpkin, winter squash

Sea vegetables: Arame, dulse, hijiki, kelp, laver, nori, wakame

Fruits: Apple, apricot, avocado, banana, berries (blackberry, blueberry, huckleberry, raspberry, strawberry) cherimoya, cherries, figs, grapes, grapefruit, kiwi, lemon, limes, loquat, mango, melons (cantaloupe, casaba, crenshaw, honeydew) orange, papaya, persimmon, peaches, pear, pineapple, plums, pomegranate, tangerine, tangelo

Oil for salads and cooking: Extra virgin olive oil, high oleic expeller pressed canola oil (available from the company Spectrum Naturals, and excellent for stir fry meals), flax oil (should always be used raw and provides the essential fatty acid linolenic acid)

Is There Room for Junk Food?

On your weight gain plan, provided that you have normal choles-terol levels and are generally in good health, some pizza or other fast food isn't going to delay your progress. It may however, zap your energy, thus preventing you from completing your exercise program included in this plan. With most things in life, moderation is the key.

Notes on Exercise

You mentioned on your health questionnaire that you don't exercise much. However, it is very important to implement a strength-training program to maximize growth. You may want to consider joining a gym or local YMCA to have access to weight machines and dumbbells. A personal trainer can assist you with performing exercises for each body part with proper form for maximum gain.

When it comes to weight training, an excellent program to follow is a split routine. The theory is to exercise each body part only one time per week, except for abs and quads (fast healing muscles). Many peo-ple who have trouble gaining weight also need to split, or separate, the days they work opposing muscle groups. For example, separating biceps from triceps can maximize growth by allowing you to really hit your reps more intensively without the negative pressure of the just trained opposing muscle group.

There is a down side to exercise for weight gain. If you are not eating enough, you will not gain weight with any exercise program. So even if you don't feel hungry, make sure to eat!

Here are some examples of split routines you might want to try:

7-Day Routine

Day 1: Chest, shoulders, triceps, abs

Day 2: Rest

Day 3: Hamstrings, calves, abs, light aerobics

Day 4: Back, abs, traps

Day 5: Rest

Day 6: Biceps, forearms, quads

Day 7: Repeat Day 1

9-Day Routine

Day 1: Chest, biceps, forearms

Day 2: Hamstrings, calves, abs

Day 3: Rest

Day 4: Back, traps, abs

Day 5: Rest

Day 6: Triceps, shoulders

Day 7: Quads, abs

Day 8: Rest

Day 9: Repeat Day 1

Alternate 9-Day Routine

Day 1: Chest, hamstrings

Day 2: Back, traps, abs

Day 3: Rest

Day 4: Triceps, shoulders, abs

Day 5: Rest

Day 6: Biceps, forearms

Day 7: Quads, calves, abs

Day 8: Rest

Day 9: Repeat Day 1

Whichever routine you decide to use, it is important to do a minimum of three sets of different exercises for each body part, per session, using a low rep, high weight format. Then mix it up every two weeks to "surprise" your muscles, preventing your body from becoming used to the program. Let's use chest as an example. Flat benching, decline benching and incline benching would equal three different exercises. In two weeks, use incline fly, seated press, cable crossovers and toss in some deep dips for good measure.

Notes on Supplementation

Altering the anabolism/catabolism balance through targeted supplementation can be a successful addition to a weight gain plan. Put simply, anabolism is the process of building tissue, and catabolism is the process of tissue breakdown.

Flax oil is used as a source of the essential macronutrient fat, plus for its anti-inflammatory components, making it an important supplement in a strength-training program. <u>Dosage</u>: Two tablespoons daily, either added to a protein shake, salad dressing or simply taken by the tablespoon.

NOTE: Never cook with flax oil. It must always be used raw and kept refrigerated.

TMX is a fantastic supplement for those trying to gain weight. It provides 42 grams of pure whey protein, 25 grams of carbohydrate and only 6 grams of sugar (from fructose). This protein shake retains a water-like consistency, which makes it invaluable for those wishing to gain weight but find that "weight gainers" induce a strong feeling of fullness, preventing them from eating the proper number of calories. The fact that TMX is very thin and water-like makes it easier to add to your plan, cutting down on some of your food intake but not interfering with your consumption of food, thus letting you comfortably reach your calorie intake needs. Furthermore, whey protein is an excellent source of protein for muscle building, and research has shown that it has anti-catabolic effects. <u>Dosage</u>: Two or three packages per day.

L-glutamine has been shown to increase growth hormone levels and support muscle development in strength trainers. <u>Dosage</u>: Four grams first thing in the morning, upon arising. Wait 20 minutes before eating.

> **NOTE:** After taking glutamine, waiting 20 minutes before eating is critical. This promotes total absorption of the product and the subsequent growth hormone release. Your powdered glutamine should contain a scoop. Each scoop contains 2 grams. Take two scoops in the morning, mixed into a glass of water. Stir with a spoon and drink immediately. About 20 minutes later, you will be able to have your TMX shake or any other breakfast that fits your lifestyle.

A **multi-vitamin** is particularly important for an individual on a weight gain program. You can acquire most essential nutrients in one single multi-vitamin. <u>Recommendation</u>: Twinlab Daily One Caps, one capsule with one meal, taken only one time during the day.

Calcium and magnesium are important for the prevention of osteo-porosis and should be taken on a daily basis, especially by women. Look for a product that contains several sources of calcium, as well as vitamin D and/or boron to aid absorption. <u>Dosage</u>:1,200 milligrams in divided doses daily.

Supplement shopping list:
> Twinlab Daily One Caps
> Jarrow L-glutamine
> Flax oil
> TMX from Biochem
> Calcium/Magnesium

You can find the suggested nutritional supplements at your local health food store or on-line. We strongly recommend that before purchasing any product that you research whether the cost, ingredients and taste suit your personal preferences and needs.

Closing Notes

Remember to use your diet pattern with the conversion chart of serving sizes specifically tailored to your diet. This will help you avoid the tedious task of counting calories.

I know all of this information seems overwhelming, rest assured that you will not have to follow as accurate a plan for the rest of your life. As time goes by, you will notice that you can easily estimate serving sizes by sight and that it is easy for you to ascertain how much you consume throughout the day with little thought.

Please print out your program until and put it up someplace where you can see it regularly. There is too much information here to remember it all. Reviewing it even for a few seconds will remind you of some bit of information that will help you stay on your new healthy routine.

APPENDIX 3

Food Journal

Name _____

Current Weight _____

Goal Weight _____

Guidelines:

Day/Time—It's important to note when you eat as well as what you eat. This helps establish trends in your eating patterns.

Food—Indicate a simple description of the food you ate.

Activity—Note where you were and/or what you were doing when you ate. This helps determine things that trigger hunger.

DAY/ TIME	FOOD	ACTIVITY	CALORIES	FAT GRAMS	CARB GRAMS	PROTEIN GRAMS

Relevant Studies

Blaak, E. Gender differences in fat metabolism. *Current Opinion in Clinical Nutrition & Metabolic Care.* 2001 Nov; 4(6):499-502.

Keys A, Taylor HL, Grande F. Basal metabolism and age of adult man. *Metabolism.* 1973 Apr;22(4):579-87.

Harris JA, Benedict FG. A biometric study of human basal metabolism. *Proc Natl Acad Sci U S A.* 1918 Dec;4(12):370-3.

Henry CJ. Basal metabolic rate studies in humans: measurement and development of new equations. *Public Health Nutr.* 2005 Oct; 8(7A):1133-52.

Horber FF, Gruber B, Thomi F, Jensen EX, Jaeger P. Effect of sex and age on bone mass, body composition and fuel metabolism in humans. *Nutrition.* 1997 Jun;13(6):524-34.

Ravussin E, Bogardus C. Relationship of genetics, age, and physical fitness to daily energy expenditure and fuel utilization. *Am J Clin Nutr.* 1989 May;49(5 Suppl):968-75.

Schofield WN. Predicting basal metabolic rate, new standards and review of previous work. *Hum Nutr Clin Nutr.* 1985;39 Suppl 1:5-41.

White CR, Seymour RS. Mammalian basal metabolic rate is proportional to body mass. *Proc Natl Acad Sci U S A.* 2003 Apr 1;100 (7):4046-9.

Chiolero A, Faeh D, Paccaud F, Cornuz J. Consequences of smoking for body weight, body fat distribution, and insulin resistance. *Am J Clin Nutr.* 2008 Apr;87(4):801-9.

Patel SR, Malhotra A, White DP, Gottlieb DJ, Hu FB. Association between reduced sleep and weight gain in women. *Am J Epidemiol.* 2006 Nov;164(10):947-54.

Fonken LK, Workman JL, Walton JC, et al. Light at night increases body mass by shifting the time of food intake. *Proc Natl Acad Sci USA.* 2010 Oct;107(43):18664-9.

Van Zant RS. Influence of diet and exercise on energy expenditure–a review. *Int J Sport Nutr.* 1992;2(1):1-19.

Ballor DL, Katch VL, Becque MD, Marks CR. Resistance weight training during caloric restriction enhances lean body weight maintenance. *Am J Clin Nutr.* 1988;47(1):19-25

Bouchez C. Make the Most of Your Metabolism. http://www.webmd.com/fitness-exercise/guide/make-most-your-metabolism. February 24, 2006.

Dulloo AG, Duret C, Rohrer D, et al. Efficacy of a green tea extract rich in catechin polyphenols and caffeine in increasing 24-h energy expenditure and fat oxidation in humans. *Am J Clin Nutr.* 1999; 70:1040–1045.

Yoshioka M, St-Pierre S, Suzuki M, Tremblay A. Effects of red pepper added to high-fat and high-carbohydrate meals on energy metabolism and substrate utilization in Japanese women. *Br J Nutr.* 1998;80(6):503-510

Lim K, Mayumi Y, Shinobu K, et al. Dietary red pepper ingestion increases carbohydrate oxidation at rest and during exercise in runners. *Med Sci Sports Exerc.* 1997;29(3):355-361.

Jo Y-H, Talmage DA, Role LW. Nicotinic receptor-mediated effects on appetite and food intake. *J Neurobiol.* 2002;53(4):618-632.

Dyck DJ. Dietary fat intake, supplements, and weight loss. *Can J Appl Physiol.* 2000;25(6):495-523.

Malaguarnera M, Cammalleri L, Gargante MP, Vacante M, Colonna V, Motta M. L-carnitine treatment reduces severity of physical and mental fatigue and increases cognitive functions in centurians: a randomized and controlled clinical trial. *Am J Clin Nutr.* 2007; 86(6):1738-44.

Villani RG, Gannon J, Self M, Rich PA. L-carnitine supplementation combined with aerobic training does not promote weight loss in moderately obese women. *Int J Sport Nutr Exerc Metab.* 2000; 10:199-207.

American Thyroid Association (ATA) Statement on "Wilson's Syndrome" 2005, Available from http://www.thyroid.org/professionals/publications/statements/99_11_16_wilsons.html

Panicker V et al. Common variation in the DIO2 gene predicts baseline psychological well-being and response to combination thyroxine plus triiodothyronine therapy in hypothyroid patients. *Journal of Clinical Endocrinology and Metabolism.* 2009, 94(5): 1623-1629.

The Action to Control Cardiovascular Risk in Diabetes Study Group. Effects of intensive glucose lowering in type 2 diabetes. *The New England Journal of Medicine.* 2008; 358: 2545-2559.

The NICE-SUGAR Study Investigators. Intensive versus conventional glucose control in critically ill patients. *The New England Journal of Medicine.* 2009; 360:1283-1297.

Bennett WL et al. Comparative effectiveness and safety of medications for type 2 diabetes: An update including new drugs and 2-drug combinations. *Annals of Internal Medicine.* 2001; 154(9): 602-613.

Medco. New study finds lack of medication compliance leads to high medical costs. Available from http://medco.mediaroom.com/index.php?s=17872&item=27749

Nissen SE, Wolski K. Effect of rosiglitazone on the risk of myocardial infarction and death from cardiovascular causes. *The New England Journal of Medicine.* 2007; 356: 2457-2471.

Vagnini F, Chilnick LD. *The weight loss plan for beating diabetes: The 5-step program that removes metabolic roadblocks, sheds pounds safely, and reverses prediabetes and diabetes.* Beverly, MA: Fair Winds Press; 2009.

Dixon JB et al. Adjustable gastric banding and conventional therapy for type 2 diabetes. *Journal of the American Medical Association.* 2008; 299(3): 316-323.

Buchwald H et al. Weight and type 2 diabetes after bariatric surgery: Systematic review and meta-analysis. *American Journal of Medicine.* 2009; 122(3): 248-256.

Garber AJ. Incretin-based therapies in the management of type 2 diabetes: rationale and reality in a managed care setting. *Am J Manag Care.* 2010;16(Suppl):S187-S194.

Holst JJ, LaSalle JR. An overview of incretin hormones. *J Fam Prac.* 2008; 57(suppl):S4-S9.

Cobble ME, Freeman JS, Garber AJ, et al. The role of incretin therapy for type 2 diabetes in family medicine. *J Fam Prac.* 2008;57(Suppl 1): S2-S31.

Jose B. Tahrani AA, Piya MK, et al. Exenatide once weekly: clinical outcomes and patient satisfaction. *Patient Pref Adhere.* 2010;4:313-324.

Drucker DJ, Buse JB, Taylor K, et al. Exenatide once weekly versus twice daily for the treatment of type 2 diabetes: a randomised, open-label, non-inferiority study. *Lancet.* 2008;372(9645):1240-1250.

Bergenstal RM, Wysham C, MacConell L, et al. Efficacy and safety of exenatide once weekly versus sitagliptin or pioglitazone as an adjunct to metformin for treatment of type 2 diabetes (DURATION-2): a randomised trial. *Lancet.* 2010;376(9739):431-439.

Kim D, MacConell L, Zhuang D, et al. Effects of once-weekly eosing of a long-acting release formulation of Exenatide on glucose control and body weight in subjects with type 2 diabetes. *Diabetes Care.* 2007; 30(6):1487-1493.

Buse JB, Drucker DJ, Taylor KL, et al. DURATION-1: Exenatide once weekly produces sustained glycemic control and weight loss over 52 weeks. *Diabetes Care.* 2010;33(6):1255-1261.

Clark JH. A critique of Women's Health Initiative studies (2002-2006). *Nucl Recept Signal.* 2006; 4:e023.

Løkkegaard E, Andreasen AH, Jacobsen RK, et al. **Hormone therapy and risk of myocardial infarction: a national register study.** *Eur Heart J.* 2008;29:2660-2668.

Chlebowski R, Kuller LH, Prentice RL, et al. Breast cancer after use of estrogen plus progestin in postmenopausal women. *N Engl J Med.* 2009; 360:573-587.

Rocca WA, Bower JH, Maraganore DM, et al. Increased risk of cognitive impairment or dementia in women who underwent oophorectomy before menopause. *Neurology.* 2007;69(11):1074-1083.

Duckles SP, Krause DN. Cerebrovascular effects of oestrogen: multiplicity of action. *Clin Exp Pharmacol Physiol.* 2007;34:801-808.

Lang LH. Estrogen replacement lowers blood pressure of older women who have hypertension. http://www.unc.edu/news/archives/mar99/estrogen.htm. March 17, 1999.

Wang C, Cunningham G, Dobs A, et al. Long-term testosterone gel (AndroGel) treatment maintains beneficial effects on sexual function and mood, lean and fat mass, and bone mineral density in hypogonadal men. *J Clin Endocrinol Metab.* 2004;89(5):2085-2098.

Malkin CJ, Pugh PJ, Jones RD, Kapoor D, Channer KS, Jones TH. The effect of testosterone replacement on endogenous inflammatory cytokines and lipid profiles in hypogonadal men. *J Clin Endocrinol Metabol.* 2004;89(7):3313-3318.

Corlett GL, Pugh PJ, Kapoor D, Jones RD, Channer KS, Jones TH. Testosterone increases interleukin 10, an anti-inflammatory cytokine, in whole blood from hypogonadal men. *Endocr Abstr.* 2002;3:252.

Cutolo M, Balleari E, Giusti M, Intra E, Accardo S. Androgen replacement therapy in male patients with rheumatoid arthritis. *Arthritis Rheum.* 1991;34:1-5.

Bizzarro A, Valentini G, Di Martino G, DaPonte A, De Bellis A, Iacono G. Influence of testosterone therapy on clinical and immunological features of autoimmune diseases assoc iated with Klinefelter's syndrome. *J Clin Endocrinol Metab.* 198; 64:32-36.

Olsen NJ, Kovacs WJ. Case report: testosterone treatment of systemic lupus erythematosus in a patient with Klinefelter's syndrome. *Am J Med Sci.* 1995;310:158-160.

Malkin CJ, Pugh PJ, Jones RD, Jones TH, Channer KS. Testosterone as a protective factor against atherosclerosis—immunomodulation and influence upon plaque development and stability. *J Endocrinol.* 2003; 178:373-380.

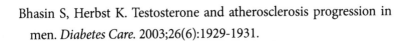

Bhasin S, Herbst K. Testosterone and atherosclerosis progression in men. *Diabetes Care.* 2003;26(6):1929-1931.

English KM, Mandour O, Steeds RP, Diver MJ, Jones TH, Channer KS. Men with coronary artery disease have lower levels of androgens than men with normal coronary angiograms. *Eur Heart J.* 2000; 21:890-894.

English KM, Steeds R, Jones TH, Channer KS. Testosterone and coronary heart disease: is there a link? *Quart J Med.* 1997;90:787-791.

Alexandersen P, Haarbo J, Christiansen C: The relationship of natural androgens to coronary heart disease in males: a review. Atherosclerosis. 1996;125:1-13.

Carroll PV, Christ ER, Bengtsson BA. Growth hormone deficiency in adulthood and the effects of growth hormone replacement: a review. Growth Hormone Research Society Scientific Committee. *J Clin Endocrinol Metab.* 1998;83(2):382-95.

van Beek AP, Wolffenbuttel BH, Runge E, Trainer PJ, Jönsson PJ, Koltowska-Häggström M. The pituitary gland and age-dependent regulation of body composition. *J Clin Endocrinol Metab.* 2010; 95(8):3664-3674.

Vance ML. Growth hormone for the elderly? *N Engl J Med.* 1990; 323: 52-54.

CPSIA information can be obtained at www.ICGtesting.com
Printed in the USA
LVOW06s1215260913

354243LV00002B/2/P